ABC of
**Ear, Nose
and Throat**

Sixth Edition

ABC series

An outstanding collection of resources for everyone in primary care

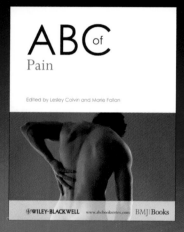

ABC of Pain

Edited by Lesley Colvin and Marie Fallon

WILEY-BLACKWELL · www.abcbookseries.com · BMJ|Books

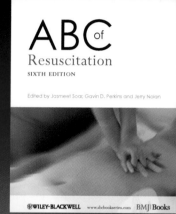

ABC of Resuscitation

SIXTH EDITION

Edited by Jasmeet Soar, Gavin D. Perkins and Jerry Nolan

WILEY-BLACKWELL · www.abcbookseries.com · BMJ|Books

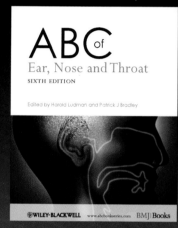

ABC of Ear, Nose and Throat

SIXTH EDITION

Edited by Harold Ludman and Patrick J Bradley

WILEY-BLACKWELL · www.abcbookseries.com · BMJ|Books

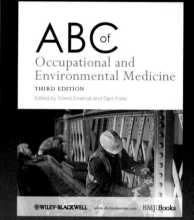

ABC of Occupational and Environmental Medicine

THIRD EDITION

Edited by David Snashall and Dipti Patel

WILEY-BLACKWELL · www.abcbookseries.com · BMJ|Books

The *ABC* series contains a wealth of indispensable resources for GPs, GP registrars, junior doctors, doctors in training and all those in primary care

▶ **Highly illustrated, informative and a practical source of knowledge**

▶ **An easy-to-use resource, covering the symptoms, investigations, treatment and management of conditions presenting in day-to-day practice and patient support**

▶ **Full colour photographs and illustrations aid diagnosis and patient understanding of a condition**

For more information on all books in the *ABC* series, including links to further information, references and links to the latest official guidelines, please visit:

www.abcbookseries.com

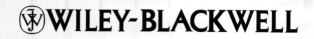

WILEY-BLACKWELL

BMJ|Books

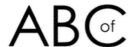

Ear, Nose and Throat

Sixth Edition

EDITED BY

Harold Ludman

Emeritus Consultant Surgeon in Otolaryngology
King's College Hospital
and
Emeritus Consultant Surgeon in Neuro-otology
National Hospital for Neurology and Neurosurgery
London, UK

Patrick J. Bradley

Honorary Professor
The University of Nottingham
and
Emeritus Consultant Head and Neck Oncologic Surgeon
Department Otorhinolaryngology – Head and Neck Surgery
Nottingham University Hospitals
Queens Medical Centre Campus
Nottingham, UK

WILEY-BLACKWELL

A John Wiley & Sons, Ltd., Publication

BMJ|Books

This edition first published 2013, © 2013 by Blackwell Publishing Ltd

BMJ Books is an imprint of BMJ Publishing Group Limited, used under licence by Blackwell Publishing which was acquired by John Wiley & Sons in February 2007. Blackwell's publishing programme has been merged with Wiley's global Scientific, Technical and Medical business to form Wiley-Blackwell.

Registered office: John Wiley & Sons Ltd, The Atrium, Southern Gate, Chichester, West Sussex, PO19 8SQ, UK

Editorial offices: 9600 Garsington Road, Oxford, OX4 2DQ, UK

The Atrium, Southern Gate, Chichester, West Sussex, PO19 8SQ, UK

111 River Street, Hoboken, NJ 07030-5774, USA

For details of our global editorial offices, for customer services and for information about how to apply for permission to reuse the copyright material in this book please see our website at www.wiley.com/wiley-blackwell.

The right of the author to be identified as the author of this work has been asserted in accordance with the Copyright, Designs and Patents Act 1988.

Library of Congress Cataloging-in-Publication Data

ABC of ear, nose, and throat / edited by Harold Ludman, Patrick J. Bradley. – 6th ed.

p. ; cm. – (ABC series)

Includes bibliographical references and index.

ISBN 978-0-470-67135-1 (pbk. : alk. paper)

I. Ludman, Harold. II. Bradley, Patrick J., 1949- III. Series: ABC series (Malden, Mass.)

[DNLM: 1. Otorhinolaryngologic Diseases. WV 140]

617.5′1–dc23

2012021107

ISBN: 9780470671351

A catalogue record for this book is available from the British Library.

Wiley also publishes its books in a variety of electronic formats. Some content that appears in print may not be available in electronic books.

Cover image: PHIL JUDE/SCIENCE PHOTO LIBRARY
Cover design by Andy Meaden

Set in 9.25/12 Minion by Laserwords Private Limited, Chennai, India
Printed in Singapore by Ho Printing Singapore Pte Ltd

1   2012

Contents

Contributors

Stephen J. Broomfield
Otology Fellow, Department of Otorhinolaryngology – Head and Neck Surgery, Nottingham University Hospitals, Queen's Medical Centre Campus, Nottingham, UK

Mered Harries
Consultant Otolaryngologist, Brighton and Sussex University Hospitals, Brighton, UK

Nick S. Jones
Professor of Rhinology, Department of Otorhinolaryngology – Head and Neck Surgery, Nottingham University Hospitals, Queen's Medical Centre Campus, Nottingham, UK

Tawakir Kamani
Specialty Registrar, Department of Otorhinolaryngology – Head and Neck Surgery, Nottingham University Hospitals, Queen's Medical Centre Campus, Nottingham, UK

Andrew H. Marshall
Consultant ENT Surgeon, Department of Otorhinolaryngology – Head and Neck Surgery, Nottingham University Hospitals, Queen's Medical Centre Campus, Nottingham, UK

Gerald W. McGarry
Consultant ENT Surgeon, Department of Otorhinolaryngology – Head and Neck Surgery, Glasgow Royal Infirmary, Glasgow, UK

William McKerrow
Consultant Otolaryngologist, Associate Postgraduate Dean, Northern Deanery, NHS Education for Scotland, Centre for Health Science, Inverness, UK

Lisha McLelland
Specialist Registrar Otorhinolaryngology, Department of Otorhinolaryngology – Head and Neck Surgery, Nottingham University Hospitals, Queen's Medical Centre Campus, Nottingham, UK

Thomasina Meehan
Consultant Audiovestibular Physician, Department of Audiovestibular Medicine, Nottingham University Hospitals, Queen's Medical Centre Campus, Nottingham, UK

Gavin A. J. Morrison
Consultant Otolaryngologist, Department of Otorhinolaryngology – Head and Neck Surgery, Guy's and St Thomas' NHS Foundation Trust, London, UK

Antony Narula
Professor in the Department of Otorhinolaryngology – Head and Neck Surgery, St Mary's Hospital, London, UK

Claudia Nogueira
Department of Otorhinolaryngology – Head and Neck Surgery, Nottingham University Hospitals, Queen's Medical Centre Campus, Nottingham, UK

Desmond A. Nunez
Head Division of Otolaryngology, University of British Columbia, Vancouver General Hospital, Vancouver, BC, Canada

Vinidh Paleri
Consultant Head and Neck Surgeon, Department of Otolaryngology – Head and Neck Surgery, Newcastle upon Tyne Hospitals, Newcastle, UK

Ricardo Persaud
Rhinology Fellow, Department of Otorhinolaryngology – Head and Neck Surgery, St Mary's Hospital, London, UK

Nick Roland
Consultant Head and Neck Surgeon, University Hospital Aintree, Liverpool, UK

Julian Rowe-Jones
Consultant Otolaryngologist & Facial Plastic Surgeon, The Nose Clinic, The Guildford Clinic, Guildford, UK

Anshul Sama
Consultant Rhinologist, Department of Otorhinolaryngology – Head and Neck Surgery, Nottingham University Hospitals, Queen's Medical Centre Campus, Nottingham, UK

Derek Skinner
Consultant ENT Surgeon / Rhinologist, Royal Shrewsbury Hospital, Shrewsbury, UK

Iain Swan
Department of Otorhinolaryngology – Head and Neck Surgery, Glasgow Royal Infirmary, Glasgow, UK

Andrew C. Swift
Consultant Rhinologist, University Hospital Aintree, Liverpool, UK

Paul Tierney
Consultant Otorhinolaryngologist, Head and Neck Surgeon, Department of Otorhinolaryngology-Head and Neck Surgery, Southmeade Hospital, Westbury-on-Trym, Bristol, UK

Patrick Walsh
Rhinology Fellow, Linacre Private Hospital, Hampton, VIC, Australia

Simon Watts
Consultant ENT and Facial Plastic Surgeon, Brighton and Sussex University Hospital, Brighton, UK

Tony Wright
Emeritus Professor of Otolaryngology, The Ear Institute, University College London, London, UK

Robin Youngs
Consultant Otolaryngologist, Gloucestershire Hospitals NHS Foundation Trust, Gloucestershire Royal Hospital, Gloucester, UK

Preface

Thirty years ago Stephen Lock, then Editor of the British Medical Journal, asked me (HL) to produce a series of articles for the journal. Subsequently these were published as the First Edition of this book (1981). He wrote of the importance of our specialty "counting for a substantial fraction of all consultations in general practice" and emphasised their economic importance. He said that the work was "collected together to provide the busy clinician with a practical, reliable source for these common problems".

Since that time the specialty of ENT has expanded, diagnostics have improved and treatment of many of diseases and disorders has changed, but the majority of patients seen in General Practice can be reassured by an accurate diagnosis and appropriate management advice. However, some patients who present with "minor or trivial" symptoms will reveal a significant diagnosis when investigated. Following treatment most will be cured, while some will suffer some functional morbidity, and others may have a serious condition that, if not treated quickly and appropriately, may result in mortality. These, the minority of patients, need to be recognised and referred quickly and appropriately for evaluation, diagnosis and treatment.

Patrick J. Bradley joined as a co-editor for the Fifth Edition (2007), and introduced several colleague specialists, recognised as experts in various subspecialties within ENT. This format has been maintained with an expansion of the topics covered.

The aims of previous editions persist in this Sixth Edition, to include a readership of medical and dental students, nurses and all the many other health workers dealing with the problems embraced by our specialty. We have rearranged the chapter titles and contents to reflect changes over recent years. The clinical practice of ENT has seen an expansion of our "workload" and now involves joint management across several disciplines: embracing neurosurgery in the handling of skull base tumours, oncology and radiotherapy for head and neck cancer, endoscopy and robotics for the surgical excision of tumours, and facial plastic surgery for the management of cosmetic and facial lesions. Current practice continues to emphasise that eradication of disease remains the priority, but the preservation or retention of function, so intimately associated with ENT, is given equal status in modern clinical and surgical practice. This edition continues to emphasise when referral for specialist diagnosis is needed, and has been brought up to date.

Harold Ludman
London
Patrick J. Bradley
Nottingham

CHAPTER 1

Examination of the Ear, Nose and Throat

Harold Ludman[1] and Patrick J. Bradley[2]

[1] King's College Hospital and National Hospital for Neurology and Neurosurgery, London, UK
[2] Nottingham University Hospitals, Queen's Medical Centre Campus, Nottingham, UK

OVERVIEW

- Taking a history of the symptoms, followed by inspection, palpation and site specific examination of the ENT should be performed in its entirety when a patient first presents with an ENT complaint

- The ability for the non-specialist to perform such an examination is limited because of lack of appropriate equipment and clinical expertise

- Examination of each site; ear, nose, mouth and neck when examined by the non-specialist should be performed in a repetitive systematic manner and the positive findings recorded, thus ensuring that should a patient represent at a later time the previous findings can be reviewed in the light of any new findings

- The specialist examination and investigation is the only *definitive* current method to ensure a definitive correct diagnosis can be made thus resulting in a correct and appropriate patient management

---

Examination

Equipment necessary

- *For the ear* – an otoscope (auriscope), comprising a handle, with battery power, light source and cone specula of various sizes and low-level magnification lens; a tuning fork vibrating at 512 kHz (lower frequencies excite vibration sense and higher ones decay too rapidly) (Figure 1.1).
- *For the nose* – Thudichum's or Killian's nasal speculae.
- For the mouth and oropharynx – Lack's tongue depressors, or spatulae (not as good, because the hand blocks the view and there is a lack of leverage)
- *For the neck* – a systematic plan is described below.
- *For all* – Good lighting; ideally from a headlight, or heard mirror and light source (Figure 1.1).
- *The larynx, pharynx (nasopharynx [or postnasal space], oropharynx and hypopharynx)* – essential parts of the specialty (Figure 1.2)

require specialist equipment, which is described in the relevant chapters.

Normal ear anatomy

The external auditory canal

The external auditory canal is 2.5 cm long in adults, extending to the tympanic membrane. The outer one-third passes through elastic

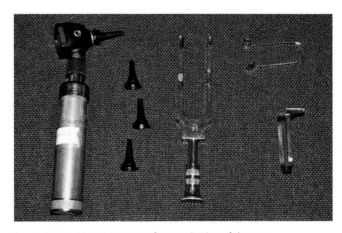

Figure 1.1 Equipment necessary for examination of the ear.

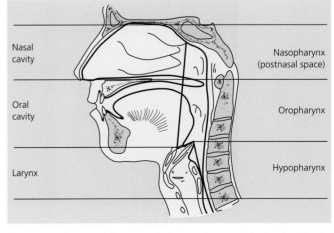

Figure 1.2 Diagram of the anatomical mucosal areas of the head and neck.

cartilage, with hair bearing skin, the inner third is through bone, with no hair and much thinner skin, adherent to the periosteum. The canal is S-shaped and must be straightened by pulling the pinna upward and backward in the adult (straight back in the child) for a better view of the tympanic membrane. The tympanic membrane lies at an angle to the canal, facing forwards and downwards, with an antero-inferior recess, where debris or foreign bodies may collect.

The tympanic membrane (TM or drumhead)

The tympanic membrane consists of a lower pars tensa and an upper pars flaccida, hiding the attic of the middle ear (Figure 1.3). The malleus handle lies in the middle layer of the pars tensa. Its handle runs downwards and backwards from a lateral process – the

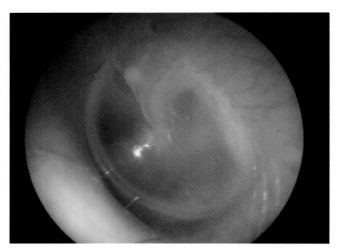

Figure 1.3 The normal tympanic membrane.

most easily recognisable structure of the drumhead at its tip (called the umbo), which is in the centre of the pars tensa. From there a cone of light – the light reflex extends antero-inferiorly.

Examination of the ear

Inspection

Compare the pinnae for symmetry.

- Examine the face for evidence of muscle weakness, as in a cranial nerve examination.
- Seek scars, from surgical or other trauma, skin inflammation, swellings, pits or sinuses around the pinna. Scars from previous surgery may be difficult to find.

Palpation

- Feel the mastoid tip, mastoid bone, the pinna itself, and also the parotid and temperomandibular joint area. Pressure on the mastoid tip and the region above and behind it must allow for any pain and tenderness of which the patient complains.

Otoscopy (with auriscope)

Choose a speculum appropriate for the patient's canal. Hold the otoscope with the hand of the same side as the ear to be examined. The otoscope should be held braced against the subject's cheek to avoid injury if the patient suddenly moves. The otoscope should be held with a 'pencil or pen grip' (as if writing), with the little finger gently touching the face, to protect against accidental over-insertion. A 'hammer' hold of the instrument is wrong (Figure 1.4a and b).

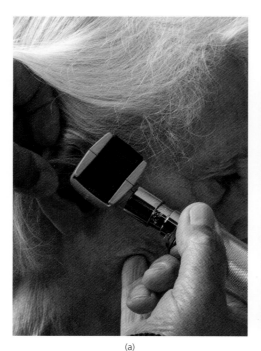

(a)

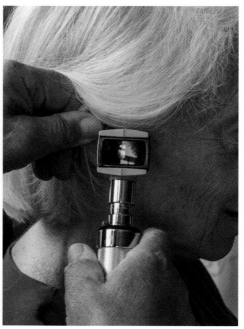

(b)

Figure 1.4 Use of an otoscope: (a) correct; (b) incorrect.

The meatus and then the tympanic membrane should be inspected systematically, with attention to all the pars tensa and the pars flaccida, which may be obscured by a crust. Most importantly, obstruction of view of the pars flaccida.

A sketch of the tympanic membrane showing any observed abnormalities is very useful.

Hearing tests

- Speech material can be used in a quiet room as a Free Field Speech Test (FFST).
- Use conversational material and so-called 'spondee' two-syllable words.
- Tuning fork tests in the non-specialist clinic include: the Rinne test and the Weber's test, which usually allow differentiation between conductive and sensorineural hearing loss.
- Pure tone audiometry and tympanometry.

Rinne test – The fork is set vibrating quietly and held adjacent to the external ear canal and then, after a few seconds, the base of the tuning fork is moved and held against the mastoid bone behind ear. The patient has been asked whether he or she can hear the sound in each position and whether it is perceived to be louder at the side of the ear canal or when placed on the mastoid bone behind the ear. A positive Rinne test result indicates that the patient heard the sound louder through the ear canal than through the mastoid bone (air conduction > bone conduction). This positive result is found if the patient has normal hearing in the test ear, or a sensorineural loss. If the patient perceives the ringing to be louder by bone conduction than through the ear canal, drum and ossicles, then there must be a fault in the conducting mechanism. In a conductive hearing loss, the Rinne test is negative (bone conduction > air conduction) (Figure 1.5). Watch out for the so-called 'false negative' Rinne test. If the patient has a very severe sensorineural deafness in one ear only, when the vibrating tuning fork is placed on the mastoid process of that side, the sound waves are transmitted through the bones of the skull to the other cochlea. The patient hears this, so that bone conduction seems louder than air conduction (which was not heard at all). This negative Rinne test does *not* indicate a conductive deafness on the side of the tested ear but is a false negative due to the totally deaf ear on that side.

Weber's test – Use a vibrating 512 kHz tuning fork placed firmly in the midline of the forehead to localise the side of the sound (see Chapter 8) (Figure 1.6). If the Weber's test is not lateralised, it indicates normal hearing or a symmetrically equal sensorineural loss. If it is lateralised to the ear with better hearing, a sensorineural loss is suggested. Lateralisation to the ear with worse hearing indicates a conductive, mechanical loss.

Tests with pure tones – To produce a **pure tone audiogram (PTA)**, for sound conducted through air and bone, require specialist facilities using an audiometer in a soundproofed room. The PTA plots the threshold of hearing at frequencies from 125 Hz to 8 kHz against the amplification in decibels needed for audibility. Air-conducted pure tones (sine waves)

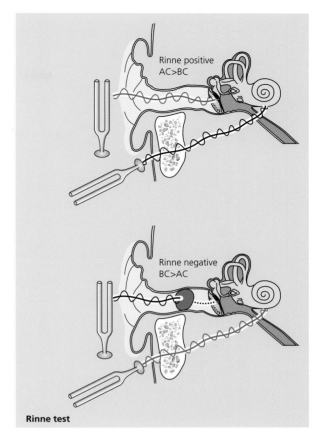

Rinne test

Figure 1.5 Rinne test.

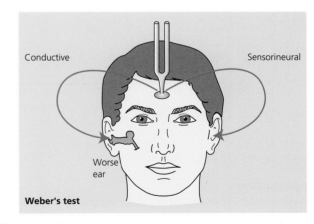

Weber's test

Figure 1.6 Weber's test.

are delivered through headphones. Bone-conducted sound is presented through a transducer held tightly against bone behind the pinna with a spring headband, while a suitable 'masking' noise is delivered to the opposite ear, to protect it from skull-transmitted signals. The audiograms obtained enable the assessment of the severity of hearing loss in each ear, and what proportion of the loss is conductive or sensorineural (Figure 1.7). Specialist texts are available that describe audiometric testing in detail.

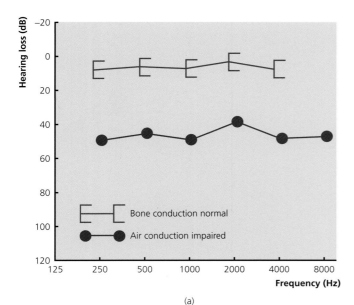

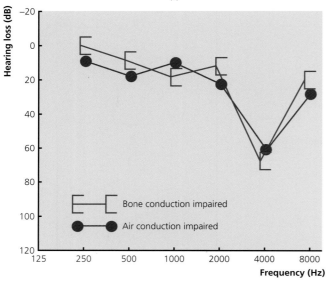

Figure 1.7 Audiograms. a) Upper shows conductive hearing loss, and b) lower sensorineural loss from noise damage.

Tympanometry

The measurement of the 'impedance' of the middle ear to conducted sound is fully described in Chapter 5.

This process can be automated by a 'tympanometer', for use in non-specialist clinics to offer a quick, *but often unreliable* suggestion of middle ear fluid – as in 'glue ear'.

Examination of the nose

Inspection

Look at the nose from the front, from either side and from above and below (see Figure 15.3).

Evaluate the size of each nostril and the nasal septum. Airway patency can be tested by placing a cold Lack's depressor underneath and asking the patient to exhale (Figure 1.8).

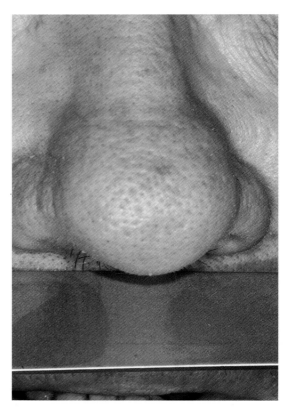

Figure 1.8 Test of nasal patency using a Lack's spatula.

Inspect the nasal cavity using an otoscope or a nasal speculum (Figure 1.9a and b) commenting on the nasal septum, the floor of the nose and the laterally placed turbinate. (If in doubt, a nasal polyp is insensitive to touch!)

Examination of the mouth

Inspection

Examine the vermilion borders of the lips.

Using a light source, preferably head mounted, ask the patient to open their mouth and protrude their tongue. Observe the width of the opening, which should be more than 2 cm allowing a two-handed examination using two Lack's tongue depressors; move the tissues about and inspect the mouth contents.

The contents should be inspected using a systematic plan. Commence superiorly with the hard and soft palate, tonsils and upper teeth, followed by the lateral mouth (the buccal mucosa), and then inferiorly with the tongue, floor of the mouth (Figure 1.10), lower teeth and lower lateral buccal area.

In a normal adult there are 32 teeth (4 'wisdom' teeth, 8 molars, 8 premolars, 4 canines and 8 incisors). When their teeth are fully erupted, children should have 20 primary teeth, which will all be replaced by permanent teeth during childhood and teens. Teeth present, absent, broken and carious should be noted and recorded.

Palpation

Palpation of the mouth floor should be bimanually from within and without, allowing the submandibular glands and the mucosa

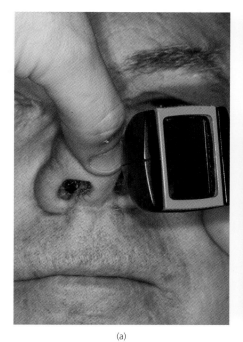

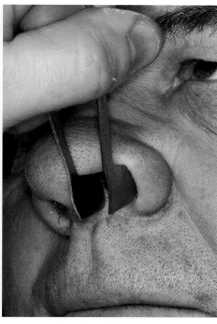

(a)

(b)

Figure 1.9 Inspection of the nasal cavity using: (a) an otoscope; (b) Thudicum's speculum.

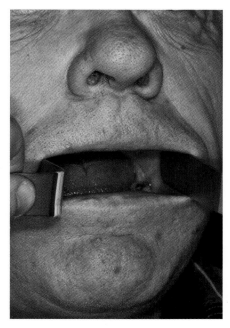

Figure 1.10 Inspection of the mouth.

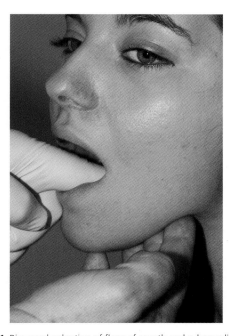

Figure 1.11 Bimanual palpation of floor of mouth and submandibular gland.

to be checked for thickening or other abnormalities, such as stones, cysts or ulcers that might suggest early cancer (Figure 1.11).

Examination of the neck

Inspection
The neck must be fully exposed from the chin above to below the level of the 'collar bones'.

Look for any swellings, skin lesions, skin discolouration, scars, etc.

Then ask the patient to identify the lump, swelling, fullness or soreness.

Any confirmed lump or lumps must be evaluated systematically by noting size, site, shape, skin (scars and colour), surface and margin, pulsation (if pulsatile, whether it is transmitted pulsation) and cross fluctuation.

Palpation
Several normal structures can be felt in the neck. In women, the cricoid cartilage is often obvious, while in men, the thyroid cartilage

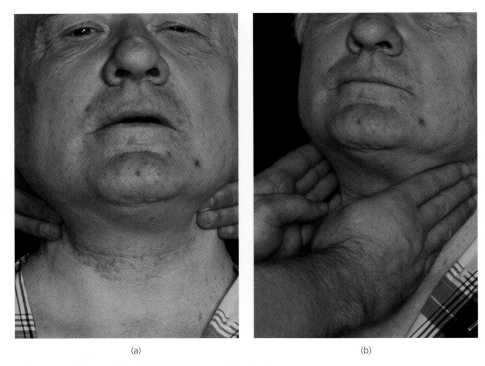

(a)   (b)

Figure 1.12 Examination of the neck: (a) correct from behind; (b) incorrect from in front.

is easily seen. The mastoid tip is readily felt behind the ear. Between the mastoid tip and the angle of the mandible, the transverse process of the C1 vertebra is sometimes palpable, especially in underweight females. The carotid bulb or bifurcation can also be felt pulsating at about the level of the hyoid bone, just beneath the sternocleidomastoid (SCM) muscle, and it can be mistaken for a mass.

The neck should be felt from behind, so that both sides can be compared (Figure 1.12a and b).

If the patient has an obvious swelling, or can point to one, then start there. Any lump should be recorded as: single or multiple, discrete or diffuse, and within a more specific list: surface, edge, temperature, consistency, fluctuation, compressibility, reducibility, pulsatility and fixation. Performing auscultation using a stethoscope may reveal a vascular bruit, but this must be done in quiet surroundings. Movement of a midline lump on the patient sticking out or the physician protruding the tongue will confirm whether the lesion is adherent to the trachea.

A systematic method for examining the neck is essential to avoid missing some areas which may later become important (Figure 1.13).

Begin at the submental area, moving along to the submandibular area. Then move from the lower pole of the parotid gland up onto the lateral parotid tissue lying on the body of the mandible up to the zygomatic arch. Onwards posteriorly to the mastoid tip, behind the ear and finally, complete the upper neck examination to include the occipital area and the cervical spine.

My practice (PJB), is to palpate the cervical spinal area down to the upper thoracic spines, extending palpation to feel the whole of the posterior triangle – tissue between the anterior border

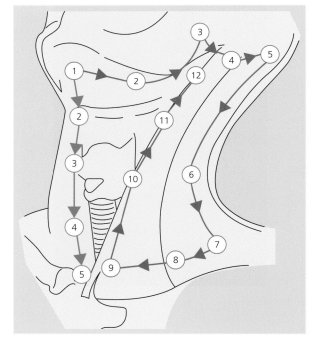

Figure 1.13 Diagram of a suggested palpation examination of the neck.

of the trapezius and the posterior border of the SCM muscle (see Figure 23.2). Palpating the supraclavicular area (from the acromioclavicular joint to the sternoclavicular joint) is followed by lateral neck palpation moving from below upwards along the anterior border of the SCM muscle to the mastoid tip.

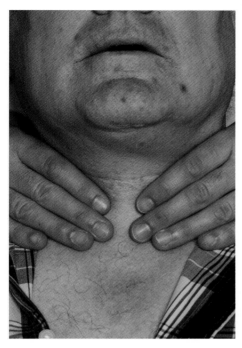

Figure 1.14 Examination of the midline of the neck.

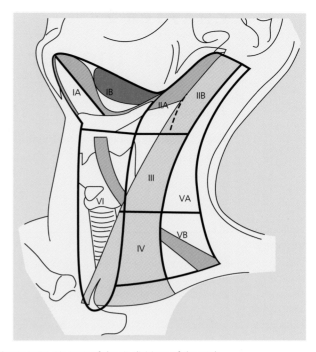

Figure 1.15 Diagram of the six divisions of the neck.

Relaxation of the SCM muscle allows one to feel deeply underneath with confidence.

The neck examination ends in the midline of the neck, from the submental area, to the hyoid, thyroid, cricoid, thyroid gland, trachea and inferiorly the sternal notch (Figure 1.14).

If a second palpation is needed, the clinician should return to that area or organ and examine that site specifically – say sub-mandibular or parotid gland, as well as the thyroid gland. The identification of a 'neck lump' in an adult may suggest a mucosal site for a potential primary malignancy. Surgical oncologists divide the neck into six regions in the neck, with three areas having subregions (Figure 1.15). The region IIa is the most frequent site presenting in clinical practice and the differential diagnosis most frequently requires a needle biopsy and a CT scan to make a firm diagnosis.

Neck examination is a supplementary examination of the throat (see earlier). In non-specialist environments, examination of the pharynx and larynx is limited, and *reliance must be placed and acted upon from symptoms*. 'Guestimation' of the seriousness of a likely cause based on symptoms alone relating to breathing, hoarseness and swallowing are statistically more likely to have a benign diagnosis than a malignancy. But the specialist examination and investigation is the only *definitive* current method to ensure a definitive correct diagnosis resulting in correct and appropriate management.

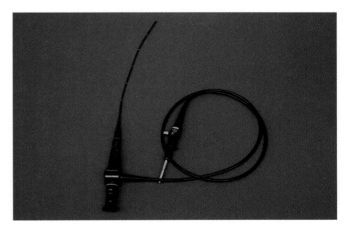

Figure 1.16 Nasendoscope used in specialist clinic to examine the pharynx and larynx.

Nasendoscopy

Examination of the nose, pharynx and larynx can be achieved without much discomfort in the majority of patients, even children, with a flexible fibre-optic instrument (Figure 1.16). It is also possible to perform more extensive evaluation of the trachea and bronchi, and oesophogoscopy with a mild sedative and topical anaesthesia (see Figure 20.3).

CHAPTER 2

Pain in the Ear

Harold Ludman

King's College Hospital and National Hospital for Neurology and Neurosurgery, London, UK

OVERVIEW

- Pain in the ear arises from ear disease, but also from non-aural disorders
- Diagnosis and management depend on skilled, experienced examination
- Other causes are only by exclusion of ear abnormalities, with reliable recognition of normality
- Referral for specialist opinion is essential whenever:
  - there is difficulty in seeing the entire meatus and tympanic membrane, or any doubt about significance of findings
  - there is suspicion of complications
- Operative intervention may be needed to confirm a diagnosis, or for treatment
- Possible complications must be suspected and treated urgently

---

Pain (otalgia, earache) is one of six symptoms that suggest ear disease (Box 2.1), these are: pain, discharge, hearing loss, tinnitus, facial weakness and vertigo.

Box 2.1 **Symptoms of ear disease**

- Pain (otalgia)
- Discharge
- Hearing loss
- Tinnitus
- Vertigo
- Facial palsy

The possible causes of otalgia are: (1) acute inflammatory processes (acute otitis externa, acute suppurative otitis media, acute coalescent mastoiditis, otitis media with effusion (OME), bullous myringitis, 'malignant' necrotising otitis externa (and some rarities); (2) referred pain; (3) neurological; (4) psychogenic (Box 2.2).

Inflammatory causes are recognized by skilled inspection of the external ear and tympanic membrane. As described in Chapter 1,

---

Box 2.2 **Causes of otalgia**

Pain in the ear (otalgia) arises from:

- acute inflammatory disease of the external ear or middle ear cleft
- diseases not primarily in the ear
  - referral from other sites
  - neurological disease
  - psychogenic

---

examination of and around the pinna, precedes that of the ear canal (external acoustic meatus) and tympanic membrane (drumhead). An otoscope is the commonest tool available in general practice (Chapter 1), but otologists always prefer the use of a headlight or head mirror with a light source to cast light in the direction of vision down the meatus, and to allow instruments to be used with both hands for the removal of wax or debris; for the assessment of drum mobility using a pneumatic speculum (which also provides low power magnification) (Figure 2.1); and to show fluid sucked through any perforation. Then the tympanic membrane is examined with a binocular microscope).

The binocular microscope (functionally similar to microscopes used in otological surgery) is essential for the fine use of microinstruments and suction apparatus, providing stereoscopic magnification of 6× or more (Figure 2.2).

If the external ear canal and the tympanic membrane are *definitely* normal (Figure 2.3), then pain is not due to ear disease. The reliability of this judgement depends entirely on the skill and experience of the examiner. Many tympanic membranes show apparent abnormalities that are not caused by acute disease. Tympanosclerotic pale yellow or white patches are an example. These are not always confidently recognised, but are irrelevant to any acute inflammatory disease. If there is any doubt, or if parts such as the attic cannot be seen, an expert otological opinion is needed (Figure 2.4).

Acute otitis externa

Acute otitis externa may be either diffuse – involving all the skin of the external meatus (Figure 2.5) or localized as a furuncle (Figure 2.6).

ABC of Ear, Nose and Throat, Sixth Edition.
Edited by Harold Ludman and Patrick J. Bradley.
© 2013 John Wiley & Sons, Ltd. Published 2013 by John Wiley & Sons, Ltd.

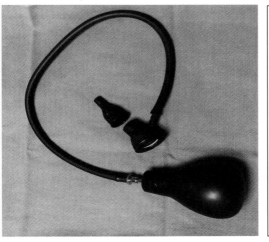

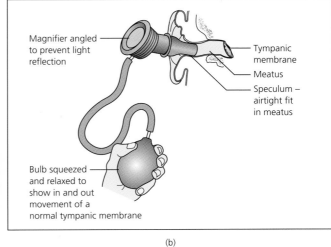

Magnifier angled to prevent light reflection

Tympanic membrane

Meatus

Speculum – airtight fit in meatus

Bulb squeezed and relaxed to show in and out movement of a normal tympanic membrane

(a)

(b)

Figure 2.1 (a) Photograph of pneumatic (Siegle's) speculum; (b) diagram of it use.

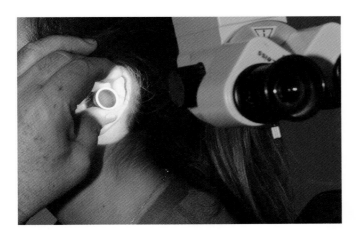

Figure 2.2 Inspection of tympanic membrane using a binocular microscope.

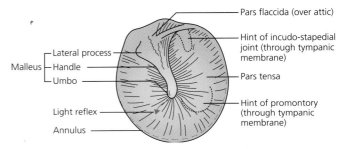

Pars flaccida (over attic)

Hint of incudo-stapedial joint (through tympanic membrane)

Lateral process

Malleus — Handle

Umbo

Pars tensa

Light reflex

Hint of promontory (through tympanic membrane)

Annulus

Figure 2.4 Labelled diagram of left tympanic membrane.

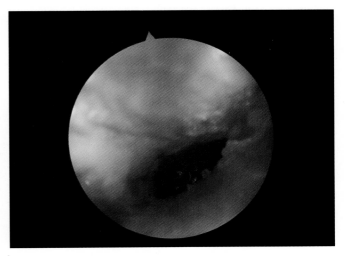

Figure 2.5 Diffuse otitis externa.

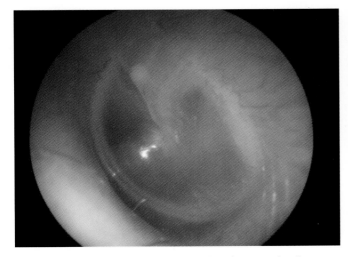

Figure 2.3 Normal left tympanic membrane: lateral process of malleus, below attic, handle of malleus with umbo at its lower end, and light reflex.

A furuncle is a tender painful swelling (a boil). It is always in the outer ear canal, where hair follicles are found, never in the inner bony meatus. Hearing is impaired only if the meatus becomes blocked by swelling or discharge, and fever occurs only if infection spreads in front of the ear, as cellulitis or erysipelas.

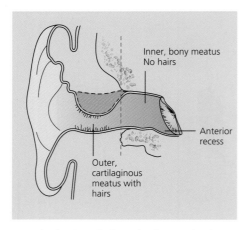

Figure 2.6 Furuncle: drawing of a furuncle of external auditory meatus.

Superficially tender enlarged nodes may be palpable in front of or behind the ear. The pinna is tender to movement in acute otitis externa, but this is never the case in acute otitis media. Discharge, if any, is usually thick and scanty, unlike the copious mucoid discharge through a tympanic membrane perforation from acute middle ear infections. Fungal skin infections cause severe pain with wet desquamation of keratin and black or coloured granules of the fruiting heads of conidiophores.

Treatment of acute otitis externa

Systemic antibiotics are only advised in acute otitis externa if there is fever or lymphadenitis. Meatal swelling is reduced by inserting a ribbon gauze wick impregnated with a deliquescent substance such as magnesium sulphate paste, or glycerine and 10% ichthammol (Figure 2.7). Proprietary expandable 'Pope' wicks (Xomed), are thin and stiff allowing careful insertion with small forceps. They soften and swell gently against the meatal walls when moistened with liquid medication. Wicks should be replaced daily until the skin swelling subsides.

Ear drops may then be used: aluminium acetate to 'toughen' the skin; 2% aceticid otic solution to restore the normal acidic state of the ear canal; or topical aminoglycoside antibiotics such as gentamicin, framycetin or neomycin, combined with corticosteroids. Topical clotrimazole is a useful antifungal agent. Systemic

analgesics, together with warmth applied through a hot pad, heat lamp, or warm oil drops, relieve pain. Any discharge should be swabbed for laboratory examination, but treatment is started before awaiting a report.

Recurrent furunculosis is always a reason to exclude diabetes.

Acute suppurative otitis media (ASOM)

Acute suppurative otitis media causes deep-seated pain, impaired hearing and systemic illness with fever. A blocked feeling in the ear, then pain and fever, are followed (usually after a few hours) by discharge when the tympanic membrane perforates – with relief of pain. The tympanic membrane shows first injection, then diffuse redness (and finally may bulge towards the examiner) (Figure 2.8); the whole middle ear cleft is affected. That is the entire air-containing space comprising the Eustachian (pharyngeal) tube, the middle ear cavity, the mastoid antrum and its adjacent mastoid air cells (Figure 2.9). For this reason, deep pressure over the mastoid antrum behind the pinna elicits tenderness in acute otitis media, but does not imply the development of mastoiditis.

Bacterial infection is usually by *Streptococcus pneumoniae*, or *Haemophilus influenzae* in very young children. Diagnosis is made

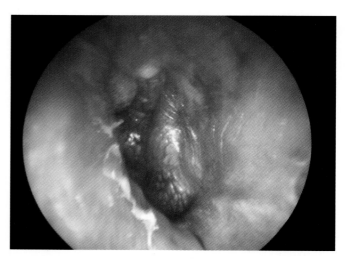

Figure 2.8 Acute suppurative otitis media: reddened tympanic membrane beginning to bulge.

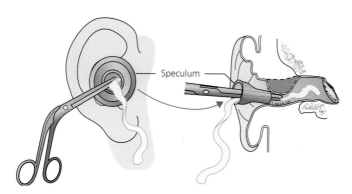

Figure 2.7 Insertion of a wick dressing.

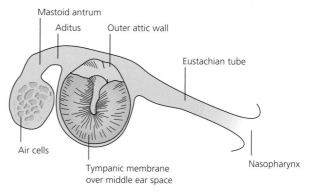

Figure 2.9 The middle ear cleft.

by inspecting the tympanic membrane, which may be prevented by wax, or by swelling from a secondary otitis externa. Only if the whole drum can be certified as normal and there is no conductive hearing loss (demonstrated by tuning fork tests with a Weber test heard centrally), can otitis media confidently be excluded. Adjacent lymph nodes are never enlarged in simple otitis media.

Treatment of acute suppurative otitis media

There is still disagreement about the need for every patient with ASOM to be treated with antibiotics, because of difficulties in analysing series in which the diagnosis has been made by groups of practitioners with varying skills in otoscopy. Without considerable experience, the condition may be diagnosed in all patients presenting with apparent redness or injection of the tympanic membrane, which is found in other conditions. It may be over-diagnosed in trials, to include patients who would recover without medication. However, the usual advice is for all suspect ASOM sufferers to be treated with systemic antibiotics – it would be impractical for all to be referred for confirmation in a specialist clinic.

The antibiotics recommended are based on likely underlying causes. The commonest infecting organisms nowadays, having displaced the very destructive Group A Streptococci, are *Streptococcus pneumoniae*, *Haemophilus influenzae* and *Moraxella catarrhalis*. The antibiotic of choice, effective against all these, is amoxicillin in doses of 125 mg t.d.s. under 2 years of age, 250 mg t.d.s. from 2 to 10 years, and 500 mg t.d.s. for older patients, or erythromycin for penicillin allergic patients (although it is less effective against *Haemophilus influenzae*, which causes 25% of cases). If β lactamase-producing organisms are likely, amoxicillin combined with clavulanic acid (as Augmentin), or trimethoprim combined with sulphamethoxazole as co-trimoxazole, is preferred. Oral administration is advised, even for the first dose (which used to be given by injection to start the course). Medication must be continued for at least 5 days. Supporting treatment includes pain relief by analgesics and warmth to the ear. Warm olive oil drops are soothing. If the tympanic membrane perforates, the ensuing discharge should be always be cultured, but an antibiotic should be changed on clinical and never solely on bacteriological grounds; however, the culture results will help to guide a change in medication, if clinical conditions suggest the need. Rarely nowadays the drum may bulge outwards under pressure without rupture, requiring urgent incision under general anaesthetic to release pus (myringotomy). This was a commonly needed procedure in the UK 50 years ago, and its need may still arise often in parts of the world where medical access is more limited than in the UK.

Recurrent acute otitis media, which is defined as three attacks within 6 months, may be provoked by predisposing causes, such as a persisting middle ear effusion, with a potentially infected accumulation of mucus persisting in the middle ear cleft. Myringotomy with insertion of a ventilation tube or 'grommet' may then be advised. Adenoid enlargement provoking repeated infection is also probably a cause; however, the role of adenoidectomy remains controversial. In the absence of predisposing factors, each attack should be treated as it arises. An alternative to consider is long-term antibiotic treatment, with ampicillin or co-trimoxazole for 3 months to 2 years.

After any episode, a return to normal is expected, and should always be confirmed clinically within 3 weeks of onset.

Acute (coalescent) mastoiditis

Acute mastoiditis is caused by the breakdown of thin bony partitions (trabeculae) between the mastoid air cells, which then become coalescent (Figure 2.10). This is a slow process that takes 2–3 weeks to develop. Throughout that time, continuing and increasingly copious discharge through a perforation in the drum persists, with general malaise and fever, unless this has been suppressed by antibiotics. If a patient has pain a few days after the tympanic membrane has been reliably judged to be normal, then that patient *cannot* have developed mastoiditis. Difficulties arise when a patient is thought to have recovered from acute otitis media, but in reality the condition has 'grumbled on' under suppression of the systemic effects with antibiotics. Mastoiditis *should* be suspected in any patient with continuous discharge from the middle ear for over 10 days, particularly if continually unwell.

The use of radiographs or, better, CT scans of the mastoid air cells helps to diagnose the condition, but not always. Only if a clearly aerated normal cell system is shown (Figure 2.11a and b) can mastoiditis be excluded. The classical appearance of breakdown of intracellular trabeculae is not always easily seen. Otitis externa may cause apparent clouding of the air cell system from oedema of soft tissues over the mastoid process. The often-described traditional classical sign of a swelling behind the ear with downward displacement of the pinna (Figure 2.12) implies a later subperiosteal abscess. This is a complication rather than a feature of mastoiditis. A subperiosteal abscess can also, by erosion of the bony outer attic wall, cause swelling in the roof of the deep part of the external ear canal, in contrast with a furuncle, which can arise only in its outer part. If any doubt persists after mastoid imaging, surgical exploration leading to a so-called 'cortical mastoidectomy' is advisable.

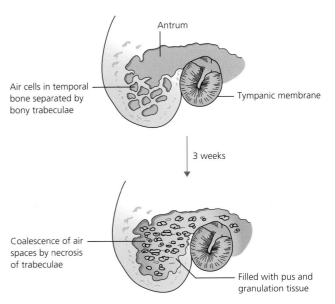

Antrum

Air cells in temporal bone separated by bony trabeculae

Tympanic membrane

3 weeks

Coalescence of air spaces by necrosis of trabeculae

Filled with pus and granulation tissue

Figure 2.10 Breakdown of the mastoid air cells.

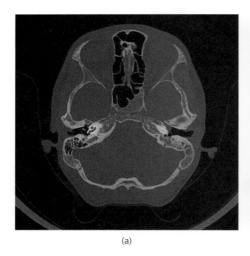
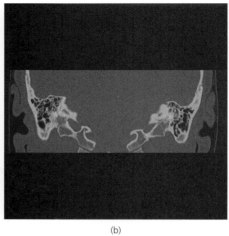

(a)   (b)

Figure 2.11 CT scan of mastoid air cells: (a) transverse CT showing mastoid air cells; (b) coronal CT, note external and internal acoustic meatus.

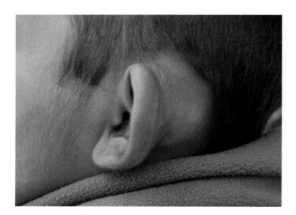

Figure 2.12 Acute coalescent mastoiditis: displacement of pinna by subperiosteal abscess.

Other complications of acute suppurative otitis media

These are all also possible complications of the bone erosive forms of chronic suppurative otitis media (Figure 2.13) (see Chapter 3). They develop if infection spreads beyond the middle ear cleft. Complications occurring *within the petrous temporal bone* include facial palsy, suppurative labyrinthitis and lateral sinus thrombophlebitis; *those occurring within the cranial cavity* are meningitis, extradural abscess, subdural abscess and brain abscess (in the temporal lobe or cerebellum).

Chronic secretory otitis media (otitis media with effusion)

Niggly, short-lived pain is a common feature of thick mucoid effusions in the middle ear air space 'glue ear'. The drum looks abnormal because of the effusion (Figures 2.14 and 2.15). Classically, there is injection with visible radial vessels, which may prompt a misdiagnosis of otitis media. The colour may be yellowish or sometimes dark blue. The child is well and afebrile however, and the associated hearing loss has usually been recognized for some time.

An essential diagnostic feature, which can be elicited by an otologist using a headlight and a pneumatic speculum, is altered mobility of the tympanic membrane. It may be totally immobile when external ear canal air pressure is raised and reduced, or there may be sluggish outward movement followed by a rapid

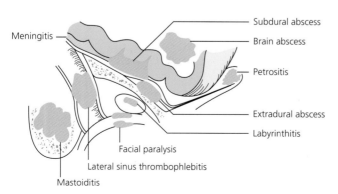

Figure 2.13 Complications of suppurative otitis media.

Meningitis

Subdural abscess

Brain abscess

Petrositis

Extradural abscess

Labyrinthitis

Facial paralysis

Lateral sinus thrombophlebitis

Mastoiditis

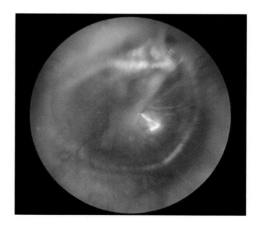

Figure 2.14 Otitis media with effusion (OME): right tympanic membrane with fluid level visible in front of handle of malleus.

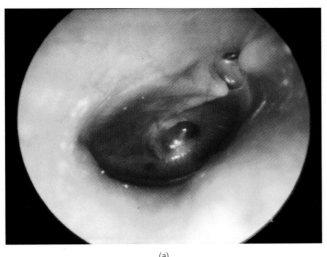
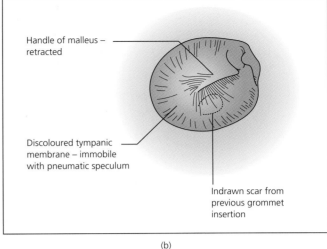

Handle of malleus –
retracted

Discoloured tympanic
membrane – immobile
with pneumatic speculum

Indrawn scar from
previous grommet
insertion

(a)   (b)

Figure 2.15 (a) Photograph of a right tympanic membrane with "glue ear"; (b) labelled diagram.

'snap' back when the partial vacuum is released. This altered mobility can also be demonstrated by tympanometry using an impedance measuring meter during continuously changing ear canal pressure, from above to below normal atmospheric level. Simple automatic tympanometers print out a quickly available chart indicating middle ear air pressure and its changes (if any) as the external ear air pressure is raised and then lowered. However, there can be technical problems in using these instruments reliably.

'Malignant' (necrotising) otitis externa

This is a rare but serious form of infection (not neoplastic, despite the unfortunate name), caused by *Pseudomonas aeruginosa* infection. It usually arises in older people with diabetes. It should be suspected if patients in this group suffer severe pain, excessive for the signs of otitis externa. Infection invades the bony base of the skull and adjacent soft tissues. Facial paralysis and other cranial nerve palsies may develop and strongly suggest the diagnosis. Mortality rates used to be high. A suspicious finding is granulation tissue in the ear canal, which must be investigated by technetium Tc-99 bone scanning. Treatment with intravenous gentamicin, with monitoring of daily blood levels, or with oral ciprofloxacin, must be administered continuously for several weeks until pain ceases, and accompanied by analgesia.

Other causes of pain

Bullous myringitis – This is another cause of severe pain. Viral (probably influenzal) infection causes haemorrhagic blistering of the eardrum (Figure 2.16) and external ear canal. There is often an associated haemorrhagic effusion in the middle ear and it may be difficult to distinguish this condition from otitis media. For that reason alone, antibiotics may be administered, but the only necessary treatment is potent analgesia.

Ramsay Hunt syndrome – Another rarity caused by varicella-zoster virus associates sudden facial palsy with a herpetic rash on the pinna (see Figure 9.1).

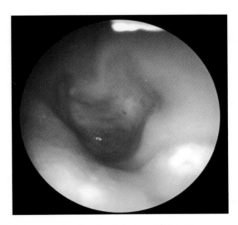

Figure 2.16 Bullous myringitis: viral infection of the ear.

Referred pain

If the external ear canal and drum are normal, with normal movement of the drum assessed with a pneumatic speculum, pain cannot be due to disease of the ear. It may well be referred from territory sharing its ultimate sensory innervation with the outer or middle ear (Figure 2.17). Pain may arise from:

- the oropharynx (IXth nerve – glossopharyngeal) in tonsillitis or carcinoma of the posterior third of the tongue
- the laryngopharynx (Xth nerve – vagus) in carcinoma of the piriform fossa
- upper molar teeth, temporomandibular joint or parotid gland (Vth nerve – trigeminal, mandibular division); Parotid causes are usually obvious; impacted wisdom teeth may not be. Temporomandibular joint problems often follow changes in bite caused by new dentures, extraction or grinding down
- the cervical spine (C2 and C3). Pain is often worse at night when the head lies awkwardly. Neck support often provides relief, as does a neck pillow under the side of the neck during sleep.

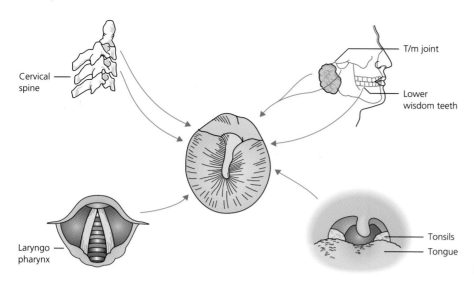

Figure 2.17 Origins of referred pain.

Neurological causes

If there is no inflammatory ear disease and no disease in sites from which pain might be referred to the ear, remaining possibilities include: glossopharyngeal neuralgia, with lancinating pain in the ear provoked by touching a trigger area within the territory of sensory innervation by the IXth cranial nerve at back of the pharynx; and migrainous neuralgia, commoner in young adult men.

Psychogenic

Often no cause can be found and pain may be attributed to depression, justifying a trial of antidepressive medication.

Further reading

Gleeson M (ed.) (2008) *Scott-Brown's Otorhinolaryngology, Head and Neck Surgery*, 7th edn, Vol. 3 (part 19): *The ear, hearing and balance*. Hodder, London.

Jerome O, Klein MD Is Acute Otitis Media a Treatable Disease? Editorial. *N Engl J Med* 2011;**364**:2.

Ludman H, Wright T (eds) (1998) *Diseases of the Ear*, 6th edn. Arnold-Hodder Headline, London.

Williams RL, Chalmers TC, Stange KC, Chalmers FT, Bowin SJ. Use of antibiotics in preventing recurrent acute otitis media and in treating otitis media with effusion: a meta-analytic attempt to resolve the brouhaha. *JAMA* 1993;**270**:1344–51.

www.nhs.uk/conditions/otitis-media

www.nhs.uk/Conditions/Otitis-externa

www.uptodate.com/contents/malignant-necrotizing-external-otitis

www.gpnotebook.co.uk/medwebpage.cfm

CHAPTER 3

Discharge from the Ear

Robin Youngs

Gloucestershire Royal Hospital, Gloucester, UK

OVERVIEW

- Discharge from the ear is an unpleasant symptom that in some communities can result in stigmatisation
- Before an accurate diagnosis can be made, the discharge should be cleared by microsuction or dry-mopping
- Topical antibiotic/steroid drops are most effective in treating otitis externa
- Discharge due to chronic otitis media occurs in the presence of a defect in the eardrum
- Cholesteatoma can be associated with serious complications

Discharge from the ear is an unpleasant symptom that reflects infection, inflammation, trauma or rarely neoplasm of the external or middle ear (Box 3.1). Persistent ear discharge and its associated odour can result in stigmatisation and social isolation in some communities (Figure 3.1).

Box 3.1 **Causes of discharging ears**

- Otitis externa (acute and chronic)
- Otitis media (acute and chronic)
- Trauma to the temporal bone
- Neoplasms of the ear (very rare)

The discharge itself arises either from the skin of the external ear canal, the surface of the tympanic membrane (eardrum), or the lining of the middle ear cleft (Figure 3.2). Discharge from the middle ear cleft often is profuse and mucoid in nature, because of the mucosal lining of the middle ear. In the clinical management of a discharging ear, accurate diagnosis is important and is facilitated by thorough history taking and examination. ENT specialists have the advantage of the use of the operating microscope available in the outpatient setting (Figure 3.3). Using the microscope in combination with suction equipment allows the specialist to aspirate

discharge and closely inspect the ear canal and tympanic membrane. In the primary care setting discharge can be removed by so-called dry-mopping using cotton wool on a suitable applicator.

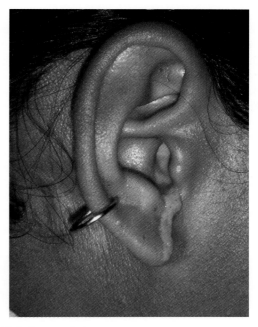

Figure 3.1 Profuse ear discharge.

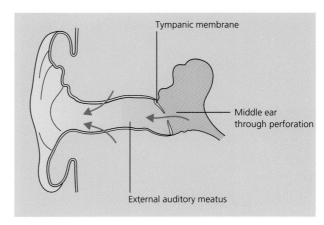

Figure 3.2 Where does discharge come from?

ABC of Ear, Nose and Throat, Sixth Edition.
Edited by Harold Ludman and Patrick J. Bradley.
© 2013 John Wiley & Sons, Ltd. Published 2013 by John Wiley & Sons, Ltd.

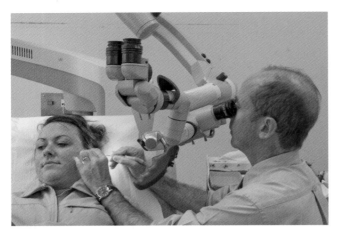

Figure 3.3 The use of the operating microscope and suction in a patient with a discharging ear.

Topical medications for discharging ears

The most useful medications for the treatment of ear discharge are delivered topically, usually in drop form, but also as ointments and creams. They contain a combination of antibiotics, antifungals, antiseptics, solvents and steroids. In this method, the ear to be treated is placed uppermost and drops instilled using the so-called displacement method. In this way pressure on the tragal cartilage forces the drops down the ear canal and, in the presence of a perforated eardrum, into the middle ear (Figure 3.4). The use of ear drops in the presence of a perforated eardrum is controversial, and centres around the use of preparations containing aminoglycoside antibiotics such as neomycin, gentamicin and framycetin. These antibiotics are particularly effective in discharging ears because they act against the Gram negative microorganisms such as *Pseudomonas aeruginosa* that are most commonly found in these conditions.

Aminoglycosides given systemically are toxic to both the auditory and vestibular parts of the inner ear. In the UK, the "data sheets" for topical aminoglycoside preparations contraindicate their use in the presence of a perforated eardrum. Nevertheless British otologists widely use aminoglycoside ear drops in treating discharging ears. The risk to the inner ear from aminoglycoside ear drops is very small indeed. Current ENT-UK guidance (Philips et al. 2007) permits their use for actively discharging ears for up to 2 weeks at a time. Other antibiotics such as quinolones (ciprofloxacin and ofloxacin) are not ototoxic and are often effective. The overuse of quinolones, however, can theoretically lead to the development of bacteria resistant to these antibiotics.

Chronic otitis externa

A number of factors predispose to the development of chronic otitis externa (Box 3.2). Normally the ear canal is kept clean by the process of epithelial migration. Desquamated skin from the deep ear canal is carried outwards where it mixes with cerumen produced by glands and is discharged from the ear canal as ear wax. Any factor that disturbs this natural process makes the development of chronic otitis externa more likely. Keen swimmers and surfers can develop bony overgrowth (exostoses) of the ear canal, which predispose to chronic infection (Figure 3.5). Trauma from the

---

Box 3.2 **Factors in the development of chronic otitis externa**

- Narrow ear canal including exostoses
- Chronic skin conditions
- Occlusion of the canal by a hearing aid or ear plug
- Frequent swimming
- Trauma to the ear canal including cotton buds
- Wax (cerumen) impaction
- Overuse of ear drops

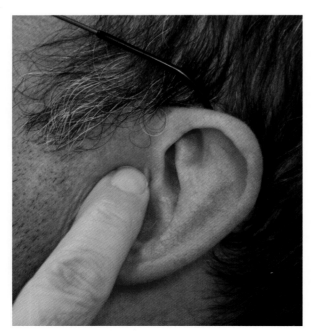

Figure 3.4 Administration of ear drops with tragal pressure.

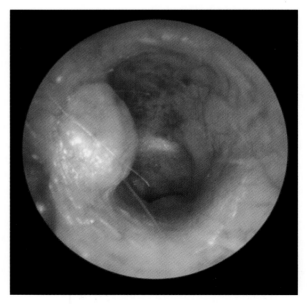

Figure 3.5 Exostoses of the external auditory canal.

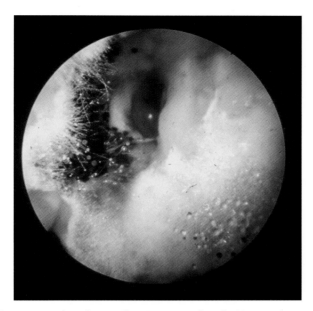

Figure 3.6 Hyphae of *Aspergillus niger* seen in fungal otitis externa.

granular myringitis, with areas of granulation tissue on the surface of the drum itself.

Preventative treatment includes avoidance of cotton buds, and water precautions when hair-washing and swimming. An effective method of preventing water ingress into the ear when hair-washing, is to use a plug of cotton wool moistened with paraffin jelly. Patients may need to avoid using a hearing aid until the condition has resolved. In the established case, treatment consists of removal of debris, followed by topical medications. Ideally debris should be removed under microscopic control. If a microscope is not available, dry-mopping with cotton wool or gentle syringing can be used. In resistant cases, a bacteriological swab to investigate the possibility of fungal infection is worthwhile. Topical steroid and antibiotic preparations can be used in drop or spray form. Fungal otitis externa usually responds to treatment with clotrimazole ear drops.

In some patients, surgical treatment may be helpful. Usually this would involve a meatoplasty procedure to widen the ear canal, particularly in the presence of canal exostoses. If a conventional hearing aid cannot be tolerated because of otitis externa then a bone-anchored hearing aid (BAHA) is an alternative.

use of cotton buds, hearing aids or other foreign bodies can damage the ear canal skin and provide a potential portal for the entry of bacteria. Skin conditions such as seborrhoeic eczema and psoriasis result in over-accumulation of keratin debris and inflammation that can become infected. The overuse of antibiotic ear drops can result in chronic fungal otitis externa (Figure 3.6).

In addition to discharge, the principle symptom of chronic otitis externa is irritation and itching of the ear canal, which may provoke further trauma. Deafness is not prominent, but can occur. Examination reveals discharge in an ear canal that is often narrowed by swelling of the canal skin (Figure 3.7). Owing to swelling of the ear canal skin and debris in the ear canal, the tympanic membrane can frequently not be seen. A variant of chronic otitis externa is

Chronic otitis media

Chronic otitis media implies a non-intact tympanic membrane allowing discharge to pass from the middle ear to the ear canal. Perforations of the tympanic membrane are described according to their anatomical location. An important landmark is the annulus of the tympanic membrane, which is the ligamentous circumferential part of the drum that inserts into the temporal bone in all but its superior part. Central perforations are in the pars tensa and are surrounded by some residual tympanic membrane or at least the annulus. The location of central perforations is denoted by their relationship to the handle of the malleus. These defects can hence be termed as anterior (Figure 3.8), posterior, inferior or subtotal. A subtotal perforation is a large perforation surrounded

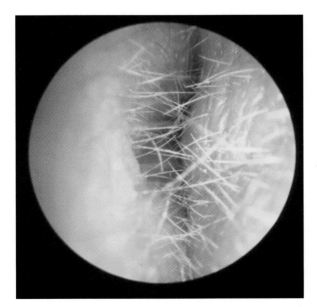

Figure 3.7 Swelling of the ear canal skin in otitis externa.

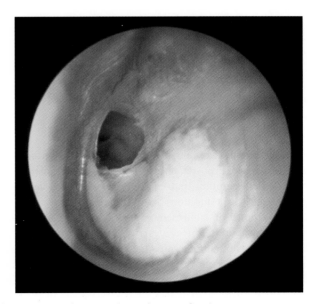

Figure 3.8 Anterior tympanic membrane perforation.

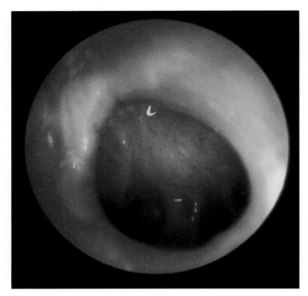

Figure 3.9 Subtotal tympanic membrane perforation.

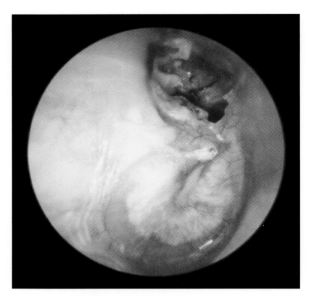

Figure 3.11 Attic perforation with cholesteatoma.

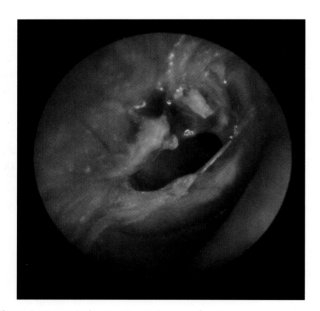

Figure 3.10 Marginal tympanic membrane perforation.

by a completely intact annulus (Figure 3.9). Marginal perforations usually occur in the posterior part of the tympanic membrane with loss of the annulus and exposure of the bony canal wall (Figure 3.10). Attic perforations occur in the superior pars flaccida part of the drum. Tympanic membrane perforations usually result from infections, but can sometimes be a result of trauma.

The symptoms of chronic otitis media are aural discharge and deafness. Deafness occurs with loss of the normal sound-conducting mechanism of the tympanic membrane and middle ear ossicles. Chronic otitis media is often associated with erosion of the incus or stapes.

Treatment of discharge in chronic otitis media consists of removal of debris from the ear canal by suction or dry-mopping, followed by topical medications.

Cholesteatoma

Attic and marginal perforations can be associated with cholesteatoma (Figure 3.11). Cholesteatoma is the abnormal accumulation of skin, squamous epithelium, within the middle ear cleft and mastoid air cells. It has the appearance of a "sac" that communicates with the ear canal (Figure 3.12) and is usually pearly white. Cholesteatoma has a tendency to progressively enlarge and can erode the bony structures of the middle and inner ear. Cholesteatoma can also spread outside the middle ear to the brain causing life-threatening complications. For this reason ears with cholesteatoma have traditionally been termed "unsafe". The complications of cholesteatoma can be grouped into intratemporal and intracranial (Table 3.1).

Surgery for chronic otitis media

Definitive treatment of discharging ears with chronic otitis media is usually surgical. These operations have a number of objectives which include stopping discharge, improving hearing and rendering an ear "waterproof" to allow bathing and swimming. In addition ears with cholesteatoma should be made "safe".

Table 3.1 Complications of cholesteatoma.

Intratemporal	Intracranial
Facial nerve paralysis	Meningitis
Lateral semicircular canal fistula	Lateral sinus thrombosis
Suppurative labyrinthitis	Extradural abscess
Subperiosteal mastoid abscess	Intracerebral abscess

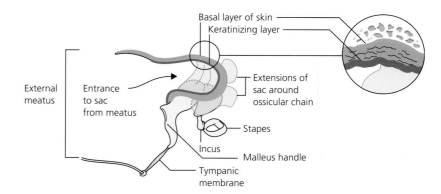

Figure 3.12 Cholsteatoma sac in attic.

Treatment of a tympanic membrane perforation without cholesteatoma usually consists of a repair of the tympanic membrane or "myringoplasty". The most used graft material is fascia taken from over the temporalis muscle through an incision behind or in front of the pinna. In addition, if the middle ear ossicles are damaged by disease an ossiculoplasty can be undertaken to improve hearing.

For ears with cholesteatoma, more extensive surgery is required. The traditional approach is to remove diseased and infected bone and to fashion a smooth, wide cavity opening into a widened external ear canal. As the ear heals the cavity becomes lined with skin and eventually becomes self cleaning through epithelial migration. Operations are named according to the extent of bone removal, which is dictated by the extent of disease.

Radical mastoidectomy is one extreme of this kind of operation. The mastoid antrum is opened with a drill and air cells opened to create a large hemispherical cavity. The incus and malleus are removed leaving only the stapes. Care is taken not to injure the facial nerve, lateral semicircular canal, sigmoid sinus and dura (Figure 3.13). Lesser operations include atticotomy, atticoantrostomy and modified radical mastoidectomy. In these operations parts of the ossicular chain and tympanic membrane may be retained or reconstructed. The surgically widened ear canal also facilitates microscopic cleaning, which in some patients has to be undertaken on a regular basis.

"Open" mastoidectomy cavities are liable to repeated infections and discharge, with swimming being avoided. Alternative operations called "combined approach tympanoplasty" aim to retain the posterior ear canal wall and hence avoid an open cavity. These so-called "closed" operations are usually undertaken in two or

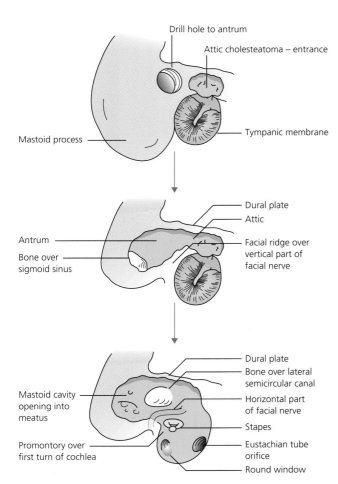

Figure 3.13 Right radical mastoidectomy.

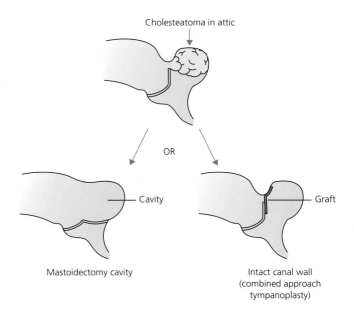

Figure 3.14 Two strategies for treating cholesteatoma.

more stages, with the second stage mainly performed to check for the presence of residual or recurrent cholesteatoma (Figure 3.14). As an open cavity is avoided, swimming is possible.

Further reading

Gleeson M (ed.) *Scott-Brown's Otorhinolaryngology, Head and Neck Surgery*, 7th edn, Vol. 3 (part 19): *The ear, hearing and balance*. Hodder Arnold, London, 2008.

Phillips JS, Yung MW, Burton MJ, Swan IR. Evidence review and ENT-UK consensus report for the use of aminoglycoside-containing ear drops in the presence of an open middle ear. *Clin Otolaryngol* 2007;**32**:330–6.

www.hawkelibrary.com. Open-access library of otoscopic images.

CHAPTER 4

Hearing Impairment in Adults

Gavin A. J. Morrison

Guy's and St Thomas' NHS Foundation Trust, London, UK

OVERVIEW

- In the UK, 6% of adults have significant hearing impairment
- Hearing impairment in adults usually occurs gradually
- Progressive loss of hearing, especially in one ear, may not be noticed by the patient
- The degree of disability depends upon the severity of the hearing loss and if it is bilateral
- Profound deafness, in one ear only, allows normal communication except when someone is speaking on that side
- A moderate bilateral high-frequency hearing impairment causes substantial problems in discriminating voices over a noisy environment
- Commonly the diagnosis can be established from a simple history and a few clinical findings: a clear view of the tympanic membranes and use of tuning fork tests

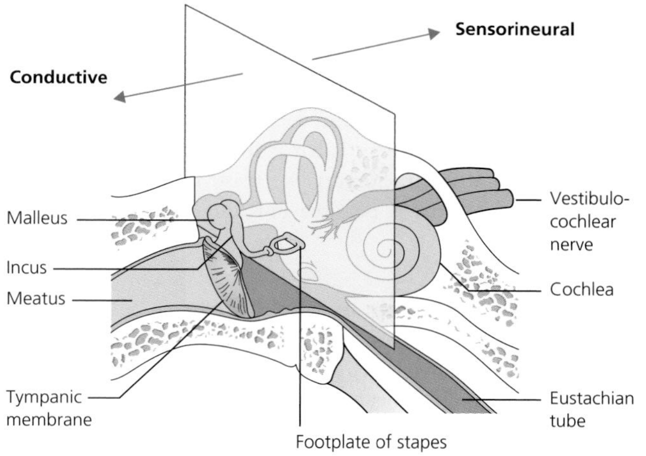

Figure 4.1 Distinction between conductive and sensorineural hearing loss.

History

Important characteristics of hearing loss are whether the onset was gradual and over what time period, whether it fluctuates, whether it is in one or both ears and how it affects the patient's quality of life. Associated symptoms might be tinnitus, dizziness or vertigo, ear ache and discharge from the ear.

Classification

Hearing loss may be categorised as conductive or sensorineural based upon the anatomical location of the problem (Figure 4.1). In conductive deafness, there is obstruction to the passage of the sound waves at any point between the outer ear and the foot plate of the stapes in the middle ear. This is the path of sound waves through the eardrum and ossicles to the cochlea. In a normally hearing ear, vibrations of the footplate of the stapes are transduced into a travelling wave within the fluids and along the basilar membrane of the cochlea. Malfunction or disease within the cochlea or auditory

nerve is termed sensorineural. In some conditions there may be a mixed hearing loss, a combination of both forms of deafness.

Conductive hearing causes

These are given in Box 4.1.

Box 4.1 **Conductive hearing loss causes**

- Wax impaction
- Otitis media with effusion (OME)
- Eustachian tube dysfunction
- Ear infections
- Perforations of the tympanic membranes
- Chronic Suppurative Otitis Media

Wax impaction

This is probably the most common cause. Frequently the patient has used cotton buds and wax becomes more deeply impacted down the ear canal. The Weber test is referred to the blocked ear. Management entails removal of the wax, by syringing in general practice or by microsuction in a specialist clinic. The use of proprietary ear drops

ABC of Ear, Nose and Throat, Sixth Edition.
Edited by Harold Ludman and Patrick J. Bradley.
© 2013 John Wiley & Sons, Ltd. Published 2013 by John Wiley & Sons, Ltd.

to soften wax for a few days beforehand is helpful. An eardrum which is known or suspected to be perforated or particularly weak should not be syringed.

Otitis externa

Inflammation of the external ear canal (otitis externa) may cause mild conductive hearing loss (Chapter 2).

Keratosis obturans

This is a condition in which there is an abnormality of normal migration of epithelium (skin) outwards along the ear canal resulting in an accumulation of desquamated keratin in the ear canal, causing blockage which needs treating by repeated microsuction and instrument clearance.

Acquired obliterative otitis externa

This follows prolonged and unsuccessful treatment of otitis externa; the ear canal scars and then the deep bony ear canal is blocked by fibrous tissue. The patient is left with a substantial conductive deafness, but a dry ear. Surgery to excise the scar and reopen and widen the meatus is possible but long-term results can be disappointing.

Tumours of the outer or middle ear

Tumours of the external or middle ear are uncommon but can present with conductive hearing loss. Any unusual looking area or non-healing ulcer of the meatal skin should be biopsied. Treatment is likely to be surgical, but malignant tumours may also require chemoradiation.

The most common middle ear neoplasm is a glomus tumour or paraganglioma. These vascular lesions present as a red swelling behind the tympanic membrane. Investigation entails specialist imaging to show the extent and probable nature of the lesion. Treatment is usually by surgical excision.

Otitis media with effusion (OME)

Persistent middle ear effusions can develop in adults with poorly functioning Eustachian tubes following upper respiratory tract infections, in the elderly, and in patients after radiotherapy to the head or skull base. Effusions are typically clear yellow. Conservative treatment includes broad-spectrum antibiotics, a short course of systemic steroids, or montelukast (leukotriene antagonist), and nasal decongestants together with attempted autoventilation of the middle ear by Valsalva manoeuvres. The nasopharynx *must* be examined endoscopically, to exclude Eustachian tube obstruction from a postnasal space lesion such as nasopharyngeal carcinoma. Non-resolving middle ear effusions can be treated surgically by insertion of ventilation tubes (grommets) in the eardrum.

Adhesive otitis media and retraction pockets

Chronic Eustachian tube dysfunction can lead to a thin (atelectatic) eardrum with retraction pockets. These may erode the ossicular chain causing hearing loss. Surgery can be helpful. Chronic inflammation of the middle ear cleft can leave a poorly aerated middle ear with scarring and adhesions (adhesive otitis media).

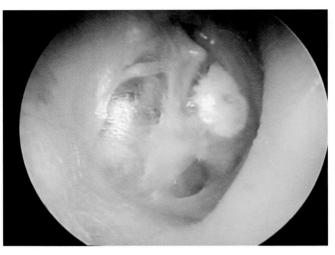

Figure 4.2 Right eardrum showing myringosclerosis anterior to handle of malleus and transparent atrophic regions.

Myringosclerosis and tympanosclerosis

Any ear in which there has been previous infection or insertion of ventilation tubes can show white or yellow scarring within the tympanic membrane known as myringosclerosis or tympanosclerosis. It does not usually cause a significant reduction in hearing (Figure 4.2). Rarely tympanosclerosis within the middle ear cleft causes scarring and fixation of the ossicles, with a conductive hearing loss.

Acute suppurative otitis media (ASOM) and chronic suppurative otitis media (CSOM)

Cases of ASOM (Chapter 2) and CSOM of either form (Chapter 3) are usually associated with conductive hearing loss. The severity will depend upon whether there is an aerated segment of middle ear and continuity of the ossicular chain. Sometimes a patient with cholesteatoma retains good hearing pre-operatively because the sound is transmitted through the cholesteatoma, after the incus has been eroded.

Surgical treatment of CSOM

Surgical treatment of CSOM is covered in Chapter 3. Among its sequelae, persistent central perforations of the tympanic membrane (Figure 4.3) can be treated by surgical repair. The indication is to stop repeated infections with discharge, to improve hearing or to allow the use of a conventional hearing aid. Surgery is successful in over 80% of patients, but carries a small risk of a permanent severe deafness. Unfit patients may often be managed by local aural toilet and topical antibiotics. Myringoplasty involves repair of the perforation, using a graft of temporalis fascia placed underneath the freshened edges of the perforation (Figure 4.4).

Ossicular defects

Erosion or discontinuity of the ossicular chain, causes a 35–40 dB conductive deafness (Figure 4.5). The diagnosis is suggested by a high compliance on the tympanogram and may be confirmed

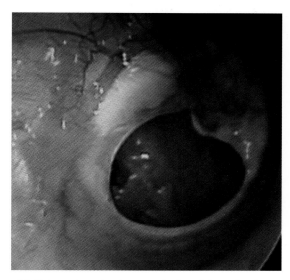

Figure 4.3 Right eardrum showing central subtotal dry perforation.

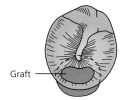

Graft

Underlay graft myringoplasty

Figure 4.4 Underlay graft myringoplasty.

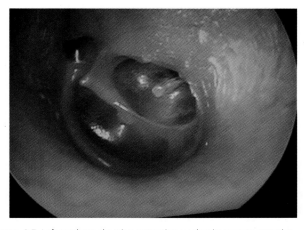

Figure 4.5 Left eardrum showing retraction pocket in postero-superior quadrant with erosion of incus. The head of the stapes and stapedius tendon are visible through the thinned posterior segment.

with a multi-planar CT scan of the ear. Management is either a hearing aid or surgery. Ossiculoplasty surgery aims to rebuild a sound conducting chain. Patients' own ossicles may be reshaped, or ossicular prostheses used.

Otosclerosis

Otosclerosis is a hereditary hearing loss caused by a localised metabolic bone disease around the otic capsule. Immature spongy bone is laid down around the footplate of the stapes bone causing fixation and a conductive deafness. The inheritance is autosomal dominant but with reduced penetrance and there may be no family history. The presentation tends to occur in young and middle aged women. It can remain unilateral or become bilateral. The presentation is usually of hearing loss of a *conductive* type and at otoscopy *there is a normal eardrum.* In the early stages a mild earache can occur.

An absence of fluoride in the water supply and previous infection with measles may be precipitating factors. Hormonal factors can accelerate progression. Pregnancy often results in deterioration, so oestrogen containing contraception should be avoided. Cochlear involvement by disease beyond the stapes footplate causes a mixed conductive and sensorineural hearing loss shown on the audiogram (Figure 4.6). Otosclerosis progresses slowly over time.

Management can be by periodic audiometry, a hearing aid or by operation. In very active disease, treatment with sodium fluoride supplements may mature the bone to a more sclerotic fixed condition, prevent further progression and render the ear more suitable for surgery.

Surgical treatment involves opening the middle ear (tympanotomy), removing the arch of the stapes bone and making a small hole in the fixed footplate so that a piston-like prosthesis can be inserted and linked to the long process of the incus (stapedotomy or stapedectomy). The surgery is successful in restoring very useful hearing in over 90% of operations (Figure 4.7). However there is a small, perhaps 1%, risk of severe permanent sensorineural loss. Successful surgery will correct the conductive deafness over the long term but will not alter the natural history for some progressive cochlear hearing loss. The indication for stapedotomy is an ear with a good prospect for correction of the conductive component, to raise hearing close to that of the other ear, and to a level where no hearing aid is required.

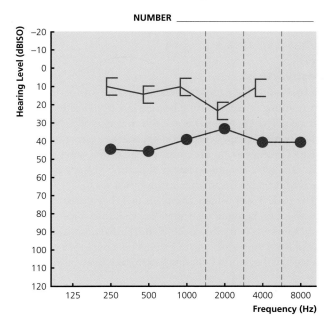

Figure 4.6 Pure tone audiogram in otosclerosis showing conductive hearing loss with 'Carhart' notch at 2000 Hz.

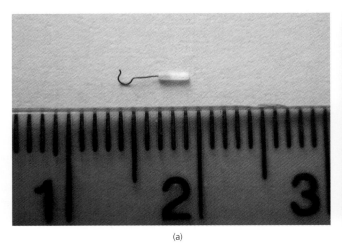

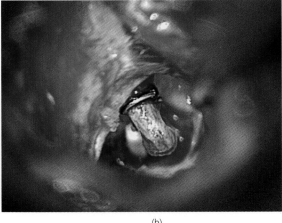

(a)

(b)

Figure 4.7 Stapedectomy surgery: (a) a smart-stapes piston; (b) piston positioned between the handle of the malleus and the footplate of the stapes.

Sensorineural hearing causes

Any adult patient who is found to have an *unexplained* hearing loss, either symmetrically in both ears, or, as is more common, with a significant asymmetry, requires imaging with an MRI scan of the internal auditory meatuses (IAMs) and posterior fossa to exclude the possibility of a vestibular schwannoma (commonly called an acoustic neuroma) in the deafer ear. (See Box 4.2 for causes of sensorial hearing loss).

Box 4.2 **Sensorineural hearing loss causes**

- Presbyacusis
- Noise-induced hearing loss
- Ménière's disease
- Hereditary hearing loss
- Drug-induced hearing loss
- Idiopathic

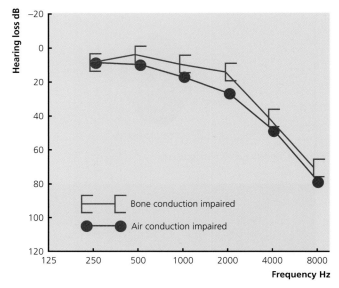

Figure 4.8 Pure tone audiogram typical of presbyacusis.

Presbyacusis

Presbyacusis is the natural process of hearing loss occurring with age, resulting in sensorineural hearing loss from death of cochlear hair cells. The age of onset is variable, but typically some hearing difficulty may be experienced from the mid 60s. Genetic factors can cause a tendency to a more advanced and earlier onset of presbyacusis. The most common pattern of hearing loss is a symmetrical one in which high frequencies are lost (Figure 4.8).

The patient will usually complain that they cannot hear easily in a noisy background or if there are multiple voices, such as at social gathering. Tinnitus can develop. The diagnosis is usually confirmed from the history, examination and a pure tone audiogram. Management comprises offering hearing aids bilaterally.

Sudden sensorineural deafness

The adult who presents with sudden sensorineural deafness, usually in one ear, should be seen and treated urgently, within a day or two of the onset. A search is made for the cause, which could

be an otologic disease such as Ménière's disease or otosclerosis, a sudden vascular event in the ear or a systemic condition such as in autoimmune vasculitis. Commonly the aetiology remains uncertain and viral infection of the inner ear or eighth nerve is presumed. Treatment is with high-dose systemic steroids started immediately. Prednisolone 60 mg per day for a week with a reducing dose over the next 10 days has been shown to increase the likelihood of spontaneous recovery. Patients are less likely to recover their hearing should starting treatment be delayed more than 24 h from the onset of ear symptoms or if initial hearing loss is severe. Investigations to look at inflammatory markers, autoimmunity and coagulopathy, as well as serial audiometry and an MRI scan to exclude a retrocochlear lesion, *must* be undertaken.

Noise-induced deafness

Exposure to noise levels louder than 85–90 dB through prolonged employment or recreation in a noisy environment, will lead to death of cochlear hair cells and usually bilateral high-tone sensorineural

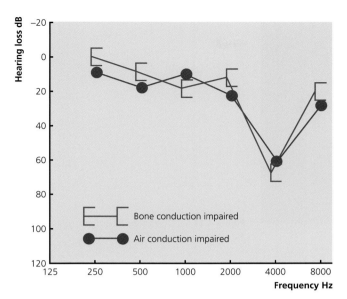

Figure 4.9 Pure tone audiogram showing 4000 Hz notch suggestive of noise damage.

deafness, initially maximal at 4000 Hz (Figure 4.9). The most susceptible groups are those using firearms or power tools such as jackhammers without adequate ear defenders, and those who are regularly exposed to excessively loud music. The presentation is often with tinnitus and bilateral hearing loss being noted in middle age, even though the original noise damage occurred in the early adult years.

Hereditary sensorineural deafness

Most hereditary sensorineural deafness is non-syndromic. It can show dominant or recessive inheritance, but the former is more common for adult-onset deafness. Often bilateral, unilateral involvement is also seen. Many causative genes have now been identified. The onset can be at any age and the audiometric pattern and rate of progression can be variable. Some patients have an audiogram that has a differing 'cookie-bite' pattern and this suggests the likely hereditary diagnosis.

Ménière's disease

Ménière's disease is discussed in Chapter 8 and is a cause of sensorineural deafness.

Drug-induced deafness

Ototoxicity is an important cause of hearing loss. The main classes of causative drugs are the aminoglycoside antibiotics and cytotoxic agents. The aminoglycosides cause sensorineural deafness ranging from high-tone loss to profound deafness. The effect is usually dose-related and daily monitoring of drug levels is important but does not prevent the problem. Rarely patients inherit a susceptibility to aminoglycoside toxicity through the maternal mitochondrial DNA. Genetic testing is possible. Often the condition being treated is life-threatening, so justifying the need for these antimicrobials.

Aminoglycoside-containing eardrops such as Sofradex, Gentisone or Otomize spray can similarly cause hearing loss if used in an ear with a perforation, especially when it is not inflamed. Treatment courses should be restricted to 7–10 days at a time to reduce the risks.

The cytotoxic agents most likely to cause sensorineural hearing loss are Taxol, platinum-based drugs and bleomycin.

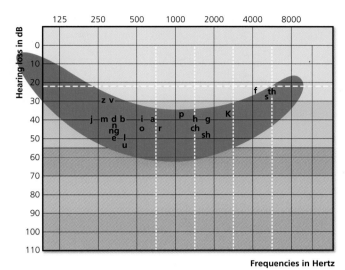

Figure 4.10 Pure tone audiogram showing the banana-shaped area surrounding the consonants at different frequencies, within which and below, there will be hearing difficulty.

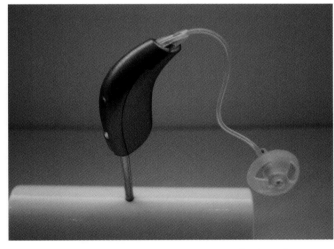

Figure 4.11 Mini-BTE open fit hearing aid (Courtesy of Cubix Ltd).

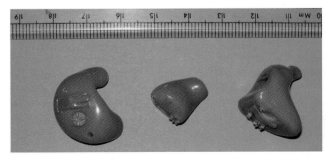

Figure 4.12 In-the-ear and in-the-canal (middle of photograph) hearing aids.

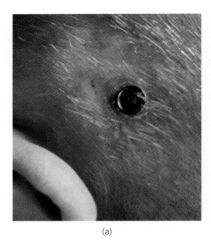
(a)

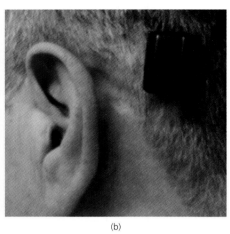
(b)

Figure 4.13 (a) Osseointegrated screw; (b) the hearing aid attached.

Other drugs associated with deafness include high doses of loop diuretics, especially with concurrent renal failure, and more reversible ototoxicity can be seen with salicylates, quinine or chloroquine-based antimalarial drugs.

Temporal bone trauma

Temporal bone trauma is discussed in Chapter 21.

Retrocochlear causes

Retrocochlear lesions cause a sensorineural deafness as a result either of obstruction to the blood supply of the labyrinth, or from direct pressure on the eighth nerve. In the posterior fossa or internal auditory meatus, the most common tumour is the benign vestibular schwannoma (acoustic neuroma). A petrous ridge meningioma can also occur at this site with similar effects. Other benign tumours of the skull base such as a glomus jugulare tumour can invade the temporal bone producing deafness and cranial nerve palsies (Chapter 6).

Central auditory processing disorders (CAP, APD)

Auditory processing disorders are most often recognised in children. In recent years, adult patients have been more commonly identified who have a functioning cochlea and reasonably normal audiometry, but have difficulty hearing. These patients may be suffering from a central auditory processing disorder. Management involves counselling and auditory training activities to enhance listening and processing skills.

Hearing aids, devices and cochlear implantation

Figure 4.10 shows a pure tone audiogram with the consonants at different frequencies, and is helpful in relating a patient's likely hearing difficulties and the probable need for a hearing aid. Conversational voice is at about 60 dB, but the primary consonants and fricatives are quieter and of high frequency. If the audiogram line falls into or below the speech banana, the patient will find it difficult to understand speech. Hearing aids can be useful for all types of hearing loss. If mid to high frequencies (2000–4000 kHz)

show hearing thresholds down to 35 dB or below, hearing aids may be helpful. However, the ability to discriminate speech can be poor in severe sensorineural hearing loss even at adequate amplification. This limits the benefit of conventional acoustic hearing aids for some patients.

A large range of digital hearing aids are available. Digital signal processing algorithms aim to optimise the benefit to users. Functions available in modern hearing aids include feedback reduction systems enabling the fitting of open moulds (useful for those who get ear infections and those who need high-frequency gain only). Teleloop settings are helpful for theatres, lectures and television. Devices differ in placement. Behind-the-ear (BTE), open fit or mini-BTE (over the ear) (Figure 4.11), in-the ear (ITE), in-the canal (ITC) (Figure 4.12) and completely in the canal (CITC) are all available.

Bone-conduction hearing aids transmit sound via a bone vibrator held against the mastoid with a band or on the arm of a pair of spectacles. They are useful for the patient who has a conductive or only moderate sensorineural deafness and when a traditional hearing aid with an ear canal insert is unsuitable.

Surgical alternatives exist for hearing with electrical devices. A bone-anchored hearing aid system (BAHA) with a titanium implant screwed into the temporal bone, onto which an external abutment is attached protruding through the skin, allows a sound processor (hearing aid) to be clipped onto it with the sound being transmitted through bone to the cochlea (Figure 4.13).

Cochlear implantation involves the surgical placement of electrodes within the cochlea to stimulate the auditory nerves directly. Implantation can be undertaken in patients with very severe or profound bilateral deafness who cannot derive benefit from acoustic hearing aids but who have a suitable cochlea and auditory nerves which can be stimulated.

Further reading

Graham J, Baguley D (eds). *Ballantyne's* Deafness, 7th edn, Wiley-Blackwell, London, 2009.

Ludman H, Wright T (eds). *Diseases of the Ear*, 6th edn, Arnold-Hodder, London, 1997.

Sataloff J, Sataloff RT (eds). *Hearing Loss*, 4th edn, Informa Healthcare, New York, 2005.

CHAPTER 5

Hearing Impairment in Children

Stephen J. Broomfield and Andrew H. Marshall

Nottingham University Hospitals, Queen's Medical Centre Campus, Nottingham, UK

OVERVIEW

- Hearing loss in children has a significant impact on quality of life
- Hearing loss in children can be conductive (most commonly glue ear), sensorineural (1 in 1000 at birth, many causes genetic/syndromic), or mixed
- In the UK, newborn hearing screening is universal. Other hearing tests in children can be subjective or objective, depending on the child's age
- Treatment of hearing loss in children can be non-surgical (e.g. provision of hearing aids) or surgical (e.g. grommet insertion, auditory implants)
- Cochlear implants have revolutionised the treatment of profound hearing loss in children

---

In children, the effects of hearing loss can be wide-ranging, affecting the development of spoken language and the quality of speech, as well as impacting on social interactions, educational achievement, behaviour, balance and safety.

Accurate diagnosis and treatment of hearing loss in children is therefore very important and relies upon close cooperation between health professionals, including audiologists, otolaryngologists, paediatricians, speech and language therapists, general practitioners, teachers (including teachers of the deaf) and health visitors.

Types of hearing loss

Hearing loss can be congenital (present at birth) or acquired (developing after birth). In either case, the hearing loss can be an isolated finding or can occur as a part of a wider neurological or developmental disorder or syndrome. Hearing loss can be conductive (related to a problem of the transmission of sound to the inner ear), sensorineural (related to a problem with the inner ear or auditory pathway) or mixed (components of both conductive and sensorineural hearing loss) (Figure 5.1). Common causes of conductive hearing loss in children are listed in Table 5.1.

ABC of Ear, Nose and Throat, Sixth Edition.
Edited by Harold Ludman and Patrick J. Bradley.
© 2013 John Wiley & Sons, Ltd. Published 2013 by John Wiley & Sons, Ltd.

Table 5.1 Causes of conductive hearing loss in children, and risk factors.

External ear	
Acquired obstruction	Wax impaction
	Foreign body
Congenital atresia	Treacher Collins syndrome
	Goldenhar syndrome
	Craniosynostoses
Middle ear	
Glue ear	Parental smoking, older siblings, day care
	Down syndrome
	Cleft palate
Ossicular abnormality	Treacher Collins syndrome
	Branchio-oto-renal syndrome
	CHARGE syndrome
	Trauma
	Cholesteatoma
	Tumours (rare)

CHARGE: Coloboma, Heart defects, choanal Atresia, Retardation of growth, Genital defects, Ear abnormalities.

Assessment of a child with hearing loss

As with other conditions, the history is vital to the assessment of the child with suspected hearing loss. In particular, enquiry should be made about risk factors for both congenital and acquired hearing loss (Tables 5.1 and 5.2). Otoscopy is the mainstay of examination, and particularly helpful in diagnosing conductive hearing loss (see later).

Diagnosis of hearing loss in children

Newborn hearing screening

In the UK, approximately 1 in 1000 children is born with severe to profound permanent hearing loss. Half of these cases have a genetic cause, with one-third of these related to a recognised syndrome (Figure 5.2).

Applied universally since 2005, the Newborn Hearing Screening Programme (NHSP) now ensures that all newborn babies have a hearing assessment performed shortly after birth. Two techniques are used:

Otoacoustic emissions (OAEs): These are sounds generated by the outer hair cells of the cochlea in response to a sound and are measured by a sensitive microphone placed in the ear canal.

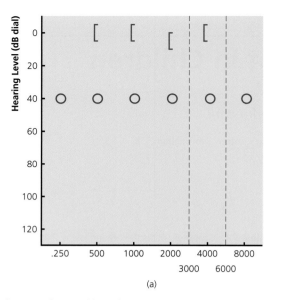
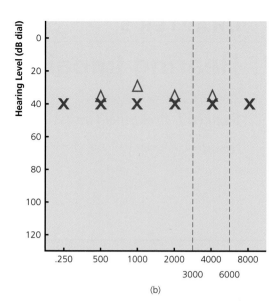

Figure 5.1 Audiograms showing (a) conductive and (b) sensorineural hearing loss. Key: Right ear: o – air conduction, [– masked bone conduction. Left ear: x – air conduction, Δ – unmasked bone conduction.

Table 5.2 Risk factors for sensorineural hearing loss in infants.

Prenatal	Family history
	Maternal alcohol/ drug use
	Infections (TORCHS)
	Ototoxic medications
Perinatal	Extreme prematurity
	Low birth weight
	Hypoxia
	Prolonged ventilation
	Sepsis
Postnatal	Infections
	Meningitis
	Other: CMV, measles, mumps
	Jaundice
	Ototoxic medications
	Head injury

TORCHS: toxoplasmosis, rubella, cytomegalovirus, *Herpes simplex*, HIV, syphilis; CMV: cytomegalovirus.

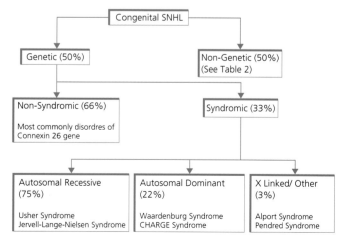

Figure 5.2 Genetics of congenital sensorineural hearing loss.

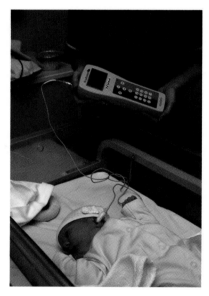

Figure 5.3 Newborn infant undergoing otoacoustic emission (OAE) test.

The test is quick and easily performed by dedicated trained screeners (Figure 5.3).

Automated auditory brainstem response (AABR): In this test, surface electrodes measure the electrical activity of the brainstem in response to an auditory stimulus. These are more accurate but also take longer than OAEs. A general anaesthetic is not required but the child must be settled, e.g. asleep or feeding.

AABR is carried out in any child who fails the OAEs test on two occasions. In addition, any baby who required admission to the special care baby unit (SCBU) or neonatal intensive care unit (NICU) has both OAEs and AABR performed, as they frequently have risk factors for hearing loss (Table 5.2).

Any baby who fails the AABR twice is referred for further assessment and early intervention.

Continued vigilance is required to ensure that no child with significant hearing loss is missed. Further screening of children in school is targeted to detect those who were missed by the NHSP or developed a progressive hearing loss.

Hearing tests in children

The method used for assessing hearing loss in children depends largely on the child's age and ability to cooperate as well as the skill and experience of the assessor, usually a paediatric audiologist. Children under the age of 6 months are generally unable to cooperate with hearing tests and therefore require objective tests such as OAEs and AABR (see above). These tests may also be useful in older children who cannot cooperate (e.g. those with neurological disorders), although such patients may need sedation or general anaesthesia.

Older children who can cooperate are suitable for behavioural audiometry, that is, hearing tests that rely on the response to a sound stimulus. Techniques include:

Visual reinforcement audiometry – Used from age 8 months to 3 years. In this test, the child sits on the parent's lap and is distracted by a tester sitting directly in front who holds their attention with a quiet activity (such as using a hand puppet). A sound is presented from the side. If the child correctly turns towards the sound, it is rewarded by a visual stimulus such as a moving toy in a box, activated by the tester. The volume and frequency of the sound can be varied to produce an accurate audiogram.

Play audiometry – Used from age 2 years. The child is first conditioned, taught to respond to a command by performing a specific task such as placing a wooden toy into a box. The child is then taught to repeat this action each time a sound is heard (Figure 5.4).

Pure tone audiometry – From age 4 or 5 years, children can often be tested using pure tone audiometry, as applied to adults.

Speech audiometry – One commonly used example is the McCormick toy test. The child is asked to identify one of 14 toys (or pictures) corresponding to a word spoken by the tester at different sound levels. The toys consist of seven pairs with similar vowel sounds, such as 'tree' and 'key'. The hearing threshold is considered to be the level at which the child correctly

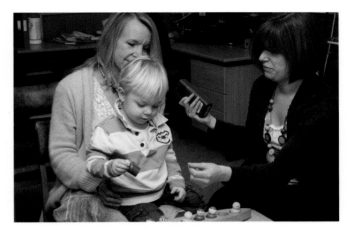

Figure 5.4 Child undergoing play audiometry.

identifies 80% of the words. This test requires some language understanding and is used from 2 years. An automated version of the test can be used as a screening tool.

In younger children, the sound for the above tests is presented in 'free field' for example using loudspeakers or spoken voice. Older children may tolerate the use of earphones or headphones, the application of sound through a bone conductor and use of a device to mask the non-test ear. This can give accurate information about each ear individually even in quite young children.

Tympanometry – This is a quick and easy test that can be applied to any age and is an important adjunct to audiometry. The machine detects the compliance of the middle ear system (ear drum and ossicular chain) by measuring how much of a sound is absorbed as the pressure is changed to above and below its normal level. In a normal ear, most sound is absorbed when the eardrum is in the normal position, i.e. when there is no pressure change. This gives a 'type A' tympanogram (Figure 5.5a). A flat trace, or 'type B' tympanogram, can occur when the eardrum fails to move, for example due to glue ear, or because there is a perforation of the eardrum (Figure 5.5b).

Otitis media with effusion

Otitis media with effusion (OME), or glue ear, is the accumulation of mucoid fluid in the middle ear, and may occur spontaneously

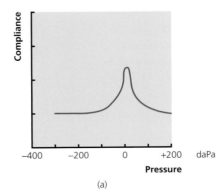
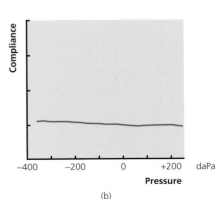

Figure 5.5 Tympanometry showing (a) type A (normal) and (b) type B (flat) traces.

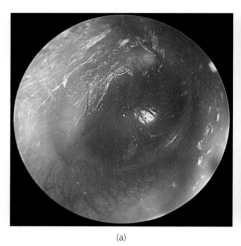
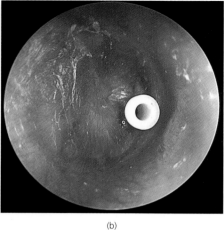

(a)   (b)

Figure 5.6 Otoendoscopic view of tympanic membrane: (a) glue ear; (b) following grommet insertion.

or following middle ear infection. Hearing is impaired to a varying degree by the reduced movement of the tympanic membrane. OME may also manifest with delayed speech development, social withdrawal, bad behaviour or imbalance. Pain is uncommon. Diagnosis is by clinical examination with audiometry and tympanometry (see above).

OME is extremely common, affecting more than 80% of children at some time before the age of 10 years, and most cases are self-limiting. Peaks in incidence occur at the ages of 2 and 5 years, and OME is more prevalent in winter. Risk factors for developing OME include having older siblings, attending day care and parental smoking. Breastfeeding is thought to be protective. Children with certain conditions, in particular Down syndrome and cleft palate, are at increased risk of developing OME.

As most cases resolve, a period of observation (known as 'watchful waiting') of 3–6 months is recommended, after which only those cases causing significant impact on the child's hearing or speech development require treatment. Various medical treatments, including antibiotics, decongestants, and steroids, have been tried but found to be ineffective. Provision of hearing aids is an option for those who do not wish to have surgery, or for those with persistent OME, including many with Down syndrome or cleft palate. More commonly, surgery is performed to drain the middle ear fluid and place a ventilation tube (grommet) in the eardrum (Figure 5.6).

This gives an immediate but temporary improvement in hearing, and the grommets extrude naturally after 9–12 months on average. Risks of grommet insertion include infection leading to otorrhoea, and chronic perforation of the tympanic membrane. Removal of the adenoid gives additional benefit when performed with grommet insertion, but the risk of postoperative bleeding must be considered. Randomised studies such as the TARGET trial, have looked at glue ear treatments, and guidelines have been produced by ENT UK and NICE.

Treatment of hearing loss

Once a hearing loss is diagnosed, the treatment will depend on its severity as well as the type of hearing loss, the cause, the child's age and the preference of the child or parents. A bilateral profound hearing loss may require urgent treatment, whereas some cases of mild or unilateral hearing loss may simply need to be observed.

Hearing aids

Hearing aids come in many forms, the commonest having a 'behind the ear' processor (Figure 5.7). They are the treatment of choice for children with sensorineural hearing loss and with modern technology can be beneficial even in cases of profound hearing loss. Some cases of conductive hearing loss may also be best treated with hearing aids.

Cochlear implants

Any child with bilateral severe to profound hearing loss who cannot be helped with optimal hearing aids may be suitable for cochlear

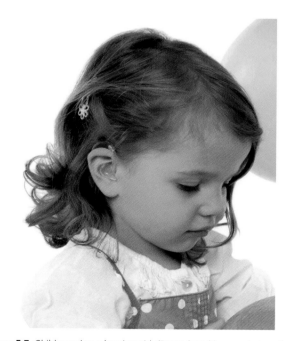

Figure 5.7 Child wearing a hearing aid. (Reproduced by permission of Phonak.)

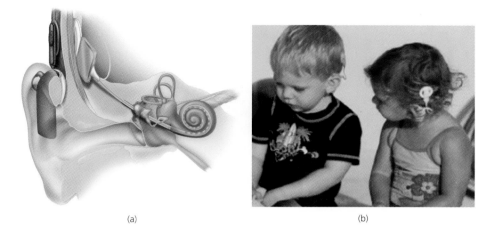

Figure 5.8 (a) Diagram illustrating cochlear implant; (b) children wearing cochlear implants. (Courtesy of Cochlear Ltd.)

(a)   (b)

implantation. A cochlear implant has both external and internal parts. The microphone and processor are worn much like a hearing aid and convert sound into an electrical signal. This is passed to the transmitter coil which attaches magnetically to a receiver coil under the scalp (Figure 5.8).

After further processing, the signal is passed down an electrode that has been surgically inserted into the cochlea, triggering an electrical signal in the auditory nerve.

Two main groups of children may benefit from cochlear implants:

A child with profound hearing loss at birth or as an infant, before learning speech, is said to be pre-lingually deaf. Newborn screening has ensured that infants born with profound hearing loss are identified early and can be referred for cochlear implantation at a young age. Infants being assessed for cochlear implantation undergo imaging of the inner ear and have paediatric, genetic and ophthalmology assessments, to exclude any co-existing abnormalities or underlying syndromes. Earlier implantation gives better results and many congenitally deaf children undergo implantation around 1 year of age. After the age of 4 years, the brain begins to lose its neuroplasticity (i.e. its ability to make new neural pathways in response to environmental stimuli) and the benefits of cochlear implantation are less predictable. Since 2009, children in the UK born profoundly deaf have been able to receive a cochlear implant for both ears, which is thought to give better directional hearing and improved understanding of sound in a noisy environment.

Children who acquire profound hearing loss after developing speech are described as post-lingually deaf. Such children must learn to interpret sounds through their implant, which can take some time. In recent years, new techniques have allowed cochlear implantation to be performed without losing residual hearing. Some children can therefore continue to use an acoustic hearing aid and a cochlear implant, so called electrical-acoustic stimulation.

Meningitis, still a common cause of post-lingual deafness despite vaccinations, can lead to inflammation which causes obliteration of the cochlear channels, making implantation impossible. Any child who has had meningitis is therefore routinely referred for a hearing test and, if required, undergoes cochlear implantation as soon as possible.

Middle ear implants

These devices may be appropriate in some children who cannot use conventional hearing aids. They may be used in mild sensorineural hearing loss as well as conductive or mixed losses. One example, the Vibrant Soundbridge, has an external processor, much like a cochlear implant. This transmits an electrical signal to the implanted device which mechanically stimulates the inner ear (Figure 5.9).

Bone-anchored hearing aids

In cases where behind-the-ear aids cannot be used, sound can be transmitted directly and very effectively to the inner ear through bone conduction. This method is particularly suitable for those with atresia of the ear canal. In younger children, a bone-conducting hearing aid is applied to the mastoid area and held in place with a headband (Figure 5.10a).

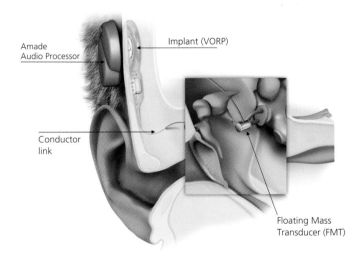

Amade
Audio Processor

Implant (VORP)

Conductor
link

Floating Mass
Transducer (FMT)

Figure 5.9 Diagram illustrating middle ear implant. (Reproduced by permission of Med-Ed.)

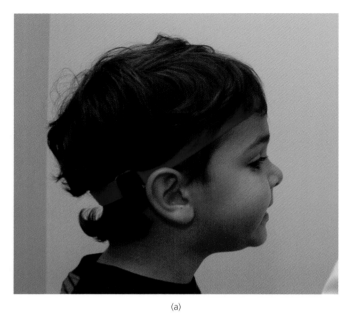
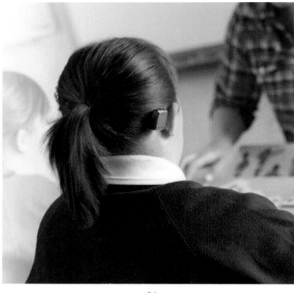

(a)
(b)

Figure 5.10 Child wearing (a) Softband bone-conducting hearing aid; (b) bone-anchored hearing aid (BAHA). (Courtesy of Cochlear Ltd.)

Older children may be suitable for surgery to fit a more permanent bone-anchored hearing aid (BAHA). Following surgery, the hearing aid is attached to the titanium screw fixture once it has knitted with the bone through a process called osseointegration (Figure 5.10b).

Other causes of hearing loss

Central processing disorders

In order to understand sounds, including speech, processing of sounds in the auditory nerve and brain is as important as inner ear function. Problems in these areas will therefore cause hearing impairment. Two specific conditions in this category are:

Auditory neuropathy – In this condition, outer hair cell function is present but there is a problem with transmission of the sound. The AABR test may be abnormal or absent. In the most severe cases, the auditory nerve may be hypoplastic or absent. In other cases the auditory nerve is anatomically normal, and the condition is therefore more correctly called auditory neuropathy/auditory dys-synchrony (AN/AD). There is a spectrum of disability caused by AN/AD, ranging from complete hearing loss to a mild impairment of hearing, often affecting the understanding of speech in background noise. Fitting of hearing aids or cochlear implantation may be appropriate, but outcomes are hard to predict.

Central auditory processing disorder – This is a group of disorders in which the peripheral hearing is normal but there is difficulty in the understanding of sound or speech due to a problem processing sound in the brain. It can be congenital or acquired, and can occur in isolation or with other central processing disorders such as autistic spectrum disorder, learning difficulties and dyslexia. Auditory training is useful in many cases, and assistance in school is often required.

Trauma

Head injury can cause conductive hearing loss (due to tympanic membrane perforation, blood in the middle ear [haemotympanum] or ossicular disruption), or sensorineural hearing loss (most commonly when a temporal bone fracture breaches the inner ear). Children with the inherited enlarged vestibular aqueduct abnormality are at particular risk of hearing loss, sometimes following a minor head injury.

Cholesteatoma

Cholesteatoma, a collection of squamous material in the middle ear or mastoid, can be congenital or acquired. As a result of cholesteatoma, ossicular disruption is common, due to erosion of the ossicular chain by the disease or removal of ossicles during surgery to eradicate the disease (see Chapter 3). Provision of hearing aids, BAHA or reconstruction of the ossicular chain (ossiculoplasty) may be required.

Further reading

ENT UK. OME (glue ear)/adenoid and grommets: position paper. 2009. www.entuk.org/position_papers/documents/OME.

Graham JM, Scadding GK, Bull PD (eds). *Pediatric ENT*. Springer, Berlin, 2007.

National Institute for Health and Clinical Excellence. Surgical management of children with otitis media with effusion (OME). 2008. http://guidance.nice.org.uk/CG60.

National Institute for Health and Clinical Excellence. Cochlear implants for children and adults with severe to profound deafness. 2009. http://guidance.nice.org/TA166.

NHS Newborn Hearing Screening Programme. http://hearing.screening.nhs.uk/

CHAPTER 6

Acoustic Neuromas and Other Cerebellopontine Angle Tumours

Tony Wright

The Ear Institute, University College London, London, UK

OVERVIEW

- Treat one-sided ear symptoms or one-sided head and neck symptoms with respect
- Whilst most tumours in the cerebellopontine angle are benign, their location is hazardous
- With the above and if the ear canal and eardrum are normal – refer
- Have a very low threshold for requesting an MRI scan
- Management options for acoustic neuromas are many and there is no single ''best'' treatment plan
- Most forms of management require long-term follow-up with careful record keeping, repeat MRI scans and review

---

The cerebellopontine angle

The cerebellopontine angle (CPA) is a tapered space between the skull and the brainstem and cerebellum, and is part of the posterior cranial fossa. It is an anatomist's dream because the boundaries of the space and the structures that run through it are many and varied and the symptoms that can arise from disease or damage to these structures are protean and can be severely disabling or in extreme fatal. The side wall of the space is the medial aspect of the petrous temporal bone housing the labyrinth. The roof is the tentorium, the tough membrane that separates the posterior cranial fossa from the middle cranial fossa. The medial wall of the space is bounded by brainstem (or pons) and the lateral lobe of the cerebellum. The CPA is filled with cerebrospinal fluid (CSF) and has important sensory and motor nerves crossing it on their way to and from the brain (Table 6.1 and Figure 6.1). A major branch of the basilar artery is the anterior inferior cerebellar artery (AICA) which courses through the CPA and itself has important branches to the pons and to the labyrinth supplying the cerebellum in part.

Running along the length of the brainstem between it and the cerebellum is the CSF-filled IVth ventricle. This has to be open to allow the circulation of the CSF and obstruction results in raised intracranial pressure and eventually an obstructive hydrocephalus.

The acoustic and vestibular nerve bundle runs across the middle of the CPA from the inner ear to the brainstem. It arises from the sensory epithelium of the cochlea and vestibular labyrinth. There is one acoustic nerve bundle but three vestibular nerve branches – superior, inferior and singular – which join and then fuse with the acoustic nerve close to the brainstem. The facial nerve runs out from the brainstem a little ahead of the acoustic and vestibular but all the nerves run through the internal auditory meatus or canal (IAM or IAC) in the petrous temporal bone (Figure 6.2). The facial nerve takes a complex path through the bone turning first forwards at the geniculate ganglion, then backwards across the middle ear, then downwards through the mastoid bone and finally forwards again through the parotid gland on its way to the muscles of facial expression (Figure 6.3) (see Chapter 9).

Growths in the CPA

With the diversity of structures in the CPA, it is not surprising that many different tumours can grow there. Fortunately, most of them are benign and by far the most common is the doubly misnamed acoustic neuroma. Not only do these usually develop on the superior vestibular nerve, but they are tumours of the nerve sheath cells – the Schwann cells – which make the myelin sheets that insulate the nerve fibres. Thus they should correctly be called vestibular schwannomas and any web search should include this term or the term neurilemmomas, which is also sometimes used by purists and pedants. They seem to arise from a single defect on the long arm of chromosome 22 which is why they rarely, if ever, become malignant, although with continued growth they can be fatal.

The incidence of acoustic neuromas has usually been quoted as 1 in 100 000 per year. With improved imaging and a greater awareness of the condition, the incidence seems to be increasing slightly. However, the post-mortem prevalence seems much higher, which suggests that many people go to their graves with these tumours rather than because of them (see "Diagnosis").

The next most common growth is a meningioma which arises from the meninges of the inner surface of the skull in this region. They are generally slow growing and of low-grade malignancy. The other lesions that can occasionally be found in the CPA are listed in Table 6.2.

A particularly unpleasant manifestation of the acoustic neuroma is as a part of the syndrome called neurofibromatosis type 2 (NF2).

ABC of Ear, Nose and Throat, Sixth Edition.
Edited by Harold Ludman and Patrick J. Bradley.
© 2013 John Wiley & Sons, Ltd. Published 2013 by John Wiley & Sons, Ltd.

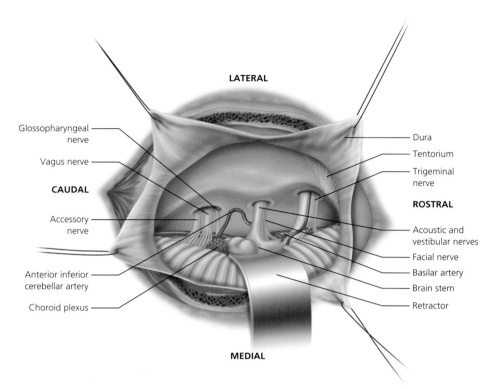

LATERAL

Glossopharyngeal nerve

Vagus nerve

CAUDAL

Accessory nerve

Anterior inferior cerebellar artery

Choroid plexus

MEDIAL

Dura

Tentorium

Trigeminal nerve

ROSTRAL

Acoustic and vestibular nerves

Facial nerve

Basilar artery

Brain stem

Retractor

Figure 6.1 Diagram of left cerebellopontine angle and its contents.

Table 6.1 Simple description of the nerves of the CPA and their major functions.

Cranial nerve	Name	Motor supply	Sensory supply	Special features
IV	Trochlear	Superior oblique moves eye down and medially		Failure causes double vision on looking down and inwards
VI	Abducent	Lateral rectus moves eye to side		Failure causes double vision on side gaze
V	Trigeminal	Chewing	Facial; scalp skin	Initial irritation causes atypical trigeminal neuralgia
VII	Facial	Facial expression	Taste: anterior $\frac{2}{3}$ tongue	Tear glands, salivary glands
VIII	Acoustic		Hearing	
VIII	Vestibular		Balance	
IX	Glossopharyngeal	Palate, swallowing	Taste: back of tongue: palate	Severe difficulty in swallowing and speaking with inhalation because of an incompetent larynx
X	Vagus	Swallowing and speech	Palate, throat	With above
XI	Accessory	Sternomastoid, trapezius		In paralysis the shoulder drops and the arm cannot be lifted properly
XII	Hypoglossal	Motor supply to the same side of the tongue		In paralysis the tongue deviates to the same side

This is an autosomal dominant condition classically presenting in youth with bilateral acoustic neuromas, other neuromas especially spinal, meningiomas and even gliomas. Fortunately this condition is rare with an estimated annual incidence of 1 in 2 355 000.

The natural history of acoustic neuromas

Some years ago, it was thought that all acoustic neuromas grew relentlessly, so that small tumours eventually became large tumours which would in turn start to compress the brainstem and cause clumsiness (ataxia) due to cerebellar malfunction. As the brainstem was further compressed, CSF circulation was compromised and raised intracranial pressure developed (see below for symptoms) before inevitable death. This process explained the need for surgical intervention in nearly all cases, despite the risks.

However, it has become clear from long-term observational studies of acoustic neuromas, that perhaps 50% or more do not grow over a 10-year period. Like many benign lesions, acoustic neuromas have a "lifespan". They start to grow, then grow at an erratic and very variable rate and eventually stop growing. The irregular growth may be because of a poor blood supply in the surrounding CSF or other intrinsic factors. Some tumours seem to continue to grow relentlessly and cause progressive symptoms, whereas others seem never to grow after diagnosis. It has recently

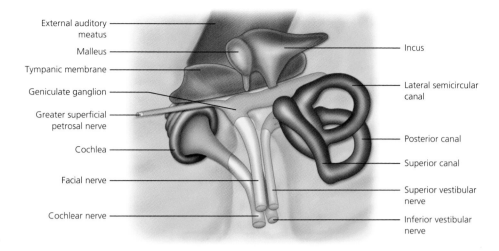

Figure 6.2 Diagram of the right petrous bone and the IAM as seen from above.

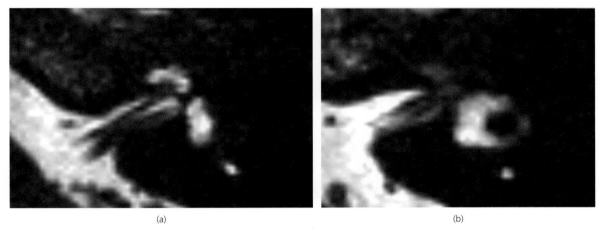

(a)   (b)

Figure 6.3 Axial MRI scan of a normal IAM with a "cut" (a) through the cochlea and showing the cochlear nerve to the left and the inferior vestibular nerve to the right; (b) through the lateral semicircular canal and showing the facial nerve to the left and the superior vestibular nerve to the right.

Table 6.2 Lesions in the CPA and their frequency of occurrence.

Type	Percentage
Acoustic Neuromas	75 at least
Meningiomas	6
Cholesteatomas	6
Gliomas	3
Others	10 at most
Metastatic tumours	
Osteomas	
Osteogenic sarcomas	
Neuromas of V, VII or IX	
Angiomas	
Papillomas of choroids plexus	
Teratomas	
Lipomas	

been found that if small intracanalicular (i.e. in the internal auditory canal) tumours do not grow over 5 years then they do not grow over a subsequent 20-year period. Unfortunately, there are currently no clues about which neuromas will grow and which have finished growing. Of those that do grow, the rate is variable but often-quoted figures are of 1–2 mm in diameter per year.

The symptoms and signs of acoustic neuromas

Many individuals with acoustic neuromas may not have any symptoms at all. Of those that do present to doctors there seem to be two groups: those that present with relatively minor otological symptoms and those that present with major neurological problems secondary to brainstem compression or the involvement of the trigeminal nerve (V) or the lower cranial nerves (IX, X, XI). Involvement of the lower cranial nerves from other neuromas or other pathologies results in a different constellation of focal symptoms, but if compression of the brainstem and IVth ventricle occurs and raised intracranial pressure develops then a generalised set of symptoms develops.

The symptoms that cause referral to an ENT surgeon are outlined in Box 6.1, and referral to a neurologist or neurosurgeon in Boxes 6.2 and 6.3. The duration of the symptoms has no relationship to the size of the tumour. The important thing is to take unilateral symptoms seriously and to investigate them. The symptoms that may result in referral to a neurologist are shown in Box 6.3 and are the result of compression of nearby structures.

Box 6.1 **Typical presenting symptoms of an acoustic neuroma seen by ENT surgeons in order of frequency**

- Unilateral alterations in hearing:
  - Distortion
  - Hearing loss
  - Tinnitus
- Unsteadiness
- One-sided headache
- Facial paraesthesia or pain
  - Atypical trigeminal neuralgia
- Deep earache
- Vertigo
- Unilateral sudden profound hearing loss.

Any one or any combination of these cardinal symptoms with a normal ear canal and eardrum warrants referral

---

Box 6.2 **Symptoms that can arise from compression of nearby structures**

- **Vth nerve:** atypical trigeminal neuralgia
- **Vth nerve:** tic douloureux
- **VII nerve:** progressive painless facial weakness
- **Brainstem:** hearing loss and tinnitus on non-tumour side
- **Xth nerve:** hoarse weak voice/dysphagia
- **XIth nerve:** dropped shoulder

Box 6.3 **Progressive symptoms arising from raised intracranial pressure**

- Clumsiness, poor balance
- Headache
- Vertigo
- Vomiting
- Fevers
- Deterioration in mental state
- Visual changes
- Fits

If the tumour is large enough to block the flow of CSF, then the generalised features of raised intracranial pressure (RICP) from an expanding space-occupying lesion in the skull become apparent and referral to a neurosurgeon frequently occurs. The features are shown in Box 6.3.

Diagnosis

Diagnosis relies on the history and examination with appropriate investigations. An ENT examination and pure tone audiogram along with an examination of the cranial nerves and cerebellar function will often suggest the possibility of a CPA mass. The next examination is an MRI scan. A T2-weighted fast spin echo (T2FSE) or turbo spin echo (T2TSE) protocol can be used to exclude or confirm a tumour whilst a gadolinium-enhanced T1 sequence will give more information about the nature of the lesion. Figures 6.4 and 6.5 show typical findings. Diffusion-weighted imaging should now also be requested in the diagnostic workup as this sequence can positively distinguish cholesteatoma from other CPA tumours.

Management

Large tumours with brainstem compression and incipient RICP

There is little disagreement about these patients who need reduction of the intracranial pressure with some form of shunt and then removal or subtotal removal of the tumour (Figure 6.6). Whether there should be total or subtotal removal depends on factors outlined below.

Small and medium-sized tumours without major neurological symptoms

Given that many tumours do not grow at all and that, even if they do grow, the rate of growth is slow, many consensus groups

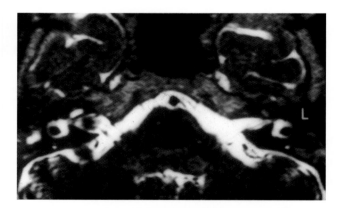

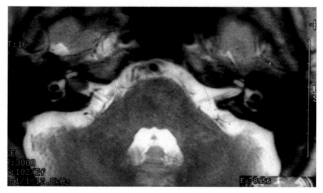

Figure 6.4 Two axial MRI scans showing small intracanalicular acoustic neuromas of the right IAM. T2- weighted scan.

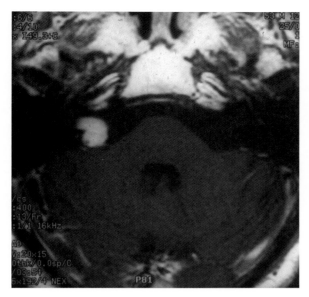

Figure 6.5 Gadolinium-enhanced T1-weighted MRI scan revealing small to medium-sized acoustic neuroma.

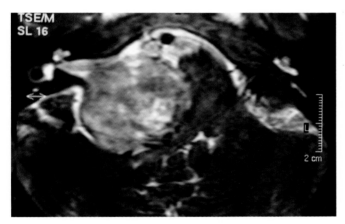

Figure 6.6 T2-weighted spin echo MRI showing large right acoustic neuroma with significant brainstem compression.

suggest that the scans should be repeated after 1 year and only if there has been growth should treatment be suggested. This requires proper discussion with the patient and relatives so that an informed decision can be made.

There are three main forms of management: watch and wait, stereotactic radiotherapy and surgery.

Watch and wait

In the elderly with small, slowly growing tumours, life expectancy may be shorter than the time that it would take the tumour to cause threatening neurological problems. A continued programme of monitoring by repeat MRI scans is sometimes recommended.

Stereotactic radiotherapy

Radiation kills tissues but a single beam directed at an acoustic neuroma is likely to kill everything in its path. Projecting multiple

small beams of radiation from different directions that are focussed on the tumour reduces the damage to surrounding tissues whilst maximising the dose in the tumour. This is called stereotactic radiotherapy (SRT). The total dose to be given is calculated from the tumour volume and then given in divided doses over 3 or 4 weeks. This is called fractionated SRT and uses X-rays. Alternatively the dose can be given in a single session. Gamma rays are usually used and the procedure is misleadingly called gamma knife treatment, and the technique radiosurgery. This is misleading because the tumour is not removed – its growth is slowed or stopped. The treatment involves a cage being fitted to the skull by small pins to ensure accurate localisation and no patient movement whilst the radiation is being administered over two or three different exposures within the single sitting. A more recent development is the cyber knife which uses X-rays but does not require a frame attached to the head and is much less claustrophobic. The risks and long-term results of this new technique are not yet catalogued.

The general risks of SRT are: (a) that it fails to work and the tumour continues to grow after which surgery is extremely difficult because of scarring; (b) there is radiation-induced damage to nearby structures – especially the facial nerve and brainstem; and (c) a long-term risk of malignant change which may make it unadvisable in the young.

Despite these reservations and although there is no tissue diagnosis, SRT is a very valuable form of treatment and is being increasingly used, despite the medium and long-term risks.

Surgery

The aim of surgery is complete removal of the tumour with no new neurological deficit. Unfortunately this is difficult to achieve with larger tumours and there is risk even with small ones. The main risk is damage to the facial nerve which is stretched around the capsule of the tumour. Even if the dissection is meticulous and the nerve is anatomically intact it sometimes fails to function. A facial paralysis is particularly distressing and anything more than minor damage (House grade 3 or more – see Chapter 9) causes a major reduction in the quality of life. The risk of a facial paralysis increases with the size of the tumour. To reduce this risk many surgeons now undertake a subtotal removal of the tumour leaving a strip of capsule on the nerve to protect it. The patient then has serial scans to detect if there is growth of the remnant. If there is, then further surgery or radiotherapy could be contemplated should the mass reach a significant size (Figures 6.7 and 6.8).

The surgical approaches are:

Transmastoid/translabyrinthine – The IAM and CPA is approached through the mastoid and, in turn, by removing the bony inner ear. This minimises traction on the brain but the hearing is lost.

Retrosigmoid/suboccipital – The craniotomy is made posterior to the sigmoid sinus and the cerebellum is retracted for access. The surgical view is as shown in Figure 6.1. With small tumours less than 1.5 cm, it may be possible to preserve the hearing. The IAC has to be opened by drilling to remove the tumour within it.

Middle cranial fossa – The craniotomy is made above the ear into the middle fossa and small intracanalicular tumours can be removed with hearing preservation. The temporal lobe has to be retracted

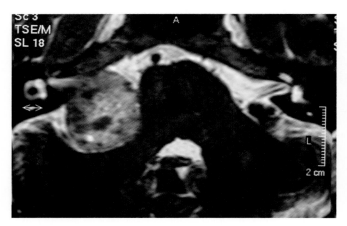

Figure 6.7 Large right-sided acoustic neuroma with some distortion of the fourth ventricle and displacement of the brainstem. Pre-operative scan.

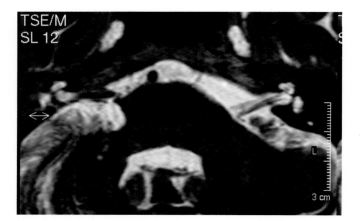

Figure 6.8 Same patient as in Figure 6.7, 1 year after surgery. There is a small area of residual neuroma/capsule on the seventh nerve. Notice how the fourth ventricle has returned to a normal shape.

for access. This approach is used less and less in Europe because of the risks of epilepsy and in the UK patients cannot drive for a year postoperatively.

Neurofibromatosis type 2

The management of this difficult condition needs a team approach with ENT surgeons and neurosurgeons working alongside hearing therapists, genetic counsellors and a social support network to deal with the problems as they arise. The MRI scan (Figure 6.9) shows large bilateral acoustic neuromas. The tumour on the right side

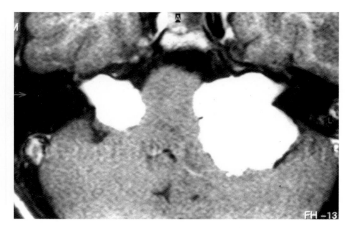

Figure 6.9 Gadolinium-enhanced MRI scan showing bilateral acoustic neuromas. That on the right has been partly removed. The patient had other intracranial and spinal tumours.

has been partly decompressed but there is now clear brainstem compression and the risk of hydrocephalus.

Summary

It is clear that there is a complexity of presentations that an acoustic neuroma can produce and that the MRI scan can reveal involvement of structures before symptoms arise. The age range of patients is wide and their individual circumstances vary greatly. There are now many forms of treatment each with advantages and drawbacks and deciding with the patient what is going to be "best" for them is not easy. There is another confounding factor exemplified by the expression: "If you only have a hammer, everything looks like a nail." The judgement of a neuro-otologic surgeon may by quite different from that of a dedicated radiotherapist, as it is influenced by their individual experience and skills, and it may not necessarily be evidence based. Until an algorithm can be constructed for a management pathway based on a good level of available evidence, then a multidisciplinary team approach may be in the individual patient's best interest despite the inherent difficulties of a multidisciplinary team.

Further reading

British Association of Otorhinolaryngologists. *Clinical Effectiveness Guidelines – Acoustic Neuromas (Vestibular Schwannoma).*, Document 5, 2002. www.orl-baohns.org

CHAPTER 7

Tinnitus

Thomasina Meehan and Claudia Nogueira

Nottingham University Hospitals, Queen's Medical Centre Campus, Nottingham, UK

OVERVIEW

- Approximately 10% of the UK population is affected by tinnitus
- Of vestibular schwannomas (acoustic neuromas), 13% present with unilateral tinnitus and have normal hearing
- Pulsatile tinnitus should be fully investigated as it may be a symptom of a cardiovascular disorder
- There are several methods designed to alleviate the distress associated with tinnitus

Tinnitus is defined as the aberrant perception of sound without any external stimulation. Tinnitus may be described as either subjective or objective. Subjective tinnitus, the most common type, occurs in the absence of any physical sound reaching the ear and is audible only to the patient. Objective tinnitus, which affects a minority of patients (1%), is generated in the body and reaches the ear through conduction in body tissue and is audible to the patient as well as the clinician (also referred to as somatosounds).

Epidemiology of tinnitus

Most people experience transient tinnitus at some time or other, particularly following exposure to loud noise. Prolonged tinnitus is experienced by approximately 10% of the adult UK population and in approximately 1% of adults, the severity of the tinnitus may severely affect their quality of life (Figure 7.1). Prevalence increases with age, although tinnitus is also commonly reported in children.

Clinical presentation

Tinnitus may be audible in one ear, both ears or in the head, and some people describe it as emanating from outside the head. Most patients report an increased awareness of tinnitus in quiet surroundings. It consists of an intermittent or continuous rushing, ringing, hissing or buzzing noise and it may be low, medium or high-pitched. The location and severity of tinnitus is not predictive of the distress experienced by the patient. Tinnitus is also commonly

ABC of Ear, Nose and Throat, Sixth Edition.
Edited by Harold Ludman and Patrick J. Bradley.
© 2013 John Wiley & Sons, Ltd. Published 2013 by John Wiley & Sons, Ltd.

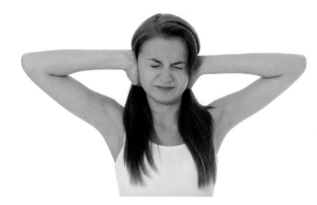

Figure 7.1 Tinnitus can have a serious impact on the quality of life. (Source: iStock © Daniel Kaesler).

associated with hyperacusis, which is characterised by a reduced tolerance to sounds at levels which would not cause discomfort in normal individuals.

Otological causes of subjective tinnitus

Tinnitus is frequently associated with hearing loss (Box 7.1) which may be conductive, sensorineural or mixed, but may also occur in individuals with normal or near-normal hearing. Hearing loss resulting from noise exposure and prebyacusis is frequently associated with tinnitus. Tinnitus may also be a feature of specific diseases such as Menière's disease. Rarely, unilateral tinnitus may be the only symptom of a vestibular schwannoma.

Box 7.1 **Pathological conditions associated with tinnitus**

- Chronic noise exposure
- Presbyacusis
- Acute acoustic trauma
- Perforation of the tympanic membrane
- Otitis media
- Menière's disease
- Vestibular schwannoma, meningioma
- Ototoxic drugs
- Whiplash injury/cochlear concussion

Subjective tinnitus and other medical conditions

Medical conditions associated with tinnitus include metal (zinc) or vitamin deficiencies, cardiovascular disorders such as a stroke, metabolic disorders such as diabetes, thyroid disease and hyperlipidaemia, and neurological disorders such as multiple sclerosis, head injuries, whiplash injuries or meningitis.

Tinnitus may also occur as a complication of certain ototoxic drugs such as non-steroidal anti-inflammatories (NSAIDs), salicylates, quinine, aminoglycosides, loop diuretics and antineoplastic drugs such as cisplatin. The ototoxic effects of NSAIDs, salicylates and quinine are dose dependent, occur at high doses and are generally reversible. Although the ototoxic effects of aminoglycosides and chemotherapeutic agents such as cisplatin are dose dependent, they can also be ototoxic at therapeutic levels, and cause permanent cochlear damage.

Other medical causes include autoimmune inner ear disease and neoplastic conditions such as a vestibular schwannoma or a meningioma.

There is a high co-morbidity between clinically significant tinnitus and anxiety and depression. Furthermore, subjects with both tinnitus and depression tend to report more severe tinnitus than those without depression.

Objective tinnitus

If the patient complains of pulsatile tinnitus, the clinician should conduct an extensive search for a skull base tumour or a vascular abnormality. There are numerous vascular causes of pulsatile tinnitus (Box 7.2); the most common being arteriovenous malformations (AVM) and fistulas. Carotid abnormalities such as atherosclerosis and aneurysms can also cause pulsatile tinnitus. Additional causes include an aberrant carotid artery, a high-riding jugular bulb and a glomus tumour. A glomus tumour may present as a red hue behind the tympanic membrane which blanches with positive pressure on carrying out pneumatic otoscopy.

Box 7.2 **Causes of objective tinnitus**

- High cardiac output
- Benign intracranial hypertension
- Dural or extracranial AV fistula
- Carotid or vertebral artery stenosis, tortuosity, dissection or aneurysm
- Aortic stenosis and mitral regurgitation
- Dural or cervical AVM
- High jugular bulb
- Vestibular schwannoma
- Temporomandibular joint syndrome
- Haemangioma
- Glomus tumour
- Otosclerosis
- Paget's disease

Benign intracranial hypertension has been reported as a major cause of pulsatile tinnitus in young women. This can be identified by papilloedema on fundoscopic examination. Systemic causes of pulsatile tinnitus include a hyperdynamic circulation due to treatment of hypertension with angiotensin converting enzyme inhibitors or calcium channel blockers. Paget's disease and otosclerosis can also cause pulsatile tinnitus, considered to be due to the neovascularisation of new bone formation, deposition and reformation.

Other causes of objective non-pulsatile tinnitus include middle ear and palatal myoclonus. Middle ear myoclonus results from activity of the stapedius and tensor tympani muscles. The sound is described as a rhythmic clicking or buzzing which is usually unilateral. Involuntary movements of the soft palate (palatal myoclonus) can cause a "clicking" tinnitus.

Pathophysiology

A useful distinction has recently been made between the ignition site of tinnitus and the mechanisms that promote the signal within the central auditory pathways. The ignition point has been defined as the site that first shows an increase in spontaneous firing rates (SFR) and is the most peripheral to do so. The site is thought to vary depending on the aetiology of the tinnitus, for example salicylate-induced tinnitus may have an ignition site within the cochlea or cochlear nerve with increased SFR within the auditory nerve fibres. Tinnitus evoked by somatic modulation such as teeth clenching may have an ignition site in the dorsal cochlear nucleus where inputs from the somatosensory system and auditory systems interact.

The physiological mechanisms responsible for tinnitus within the central auditory pathways include an increase in spontaneous discharge rates, an imbalance between excitation and inhibition with a release of excitatory inputs and reorganisation of the central auditory pathways.

Clinical assessment

There are no known objective tests that can determine the severity of subjective tinnitus.

A detailed case history is important to determine the type and characteristics of tinnitus: for example pulsatile or non-pulsatile, unilateral, bilateral or in the head, intermittent or continuous and masking by environmental noise. One should enquire about the onset, duration and potential causal relationship and trigger mechanisms such as previous noise exposure, associated hearing difficulties, hyperacusis and history of vertigo. The clinician should also enquire about the occupational status of the patient and establish how much trouble the patient is having in terms of sleep disturbance, impaired concentration, psychoemotional and psychosocial issues, as this will dictate whether and how much treatment is necessary.

Clinical examination and investigations

The following examination and investigations are suggested.

- Otoscopy (Figure 7.2)
- Tuning fork tests to uncover a conductive or sensorineural hearing loss (Figure 7.3)

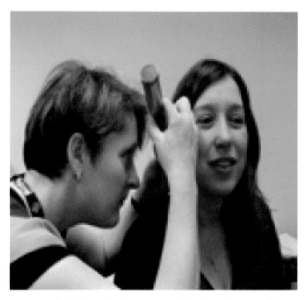

Figure 7.2 Otological examination is essential in the evaluation of tinnitus.

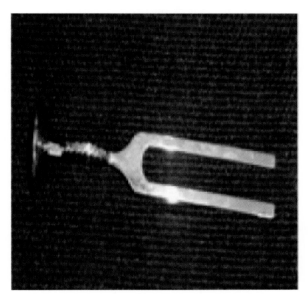

Figure 7.3 A tuning fork is used for the diagnosis of a conductive or a sensorineural hearing loss.

- Auscultation of the ear canal, preauricular and postauricular regions, orbit and neck for a carotid bruit, jugular venous hum, AVM thrill or myoclonic clicks (Figure 7.4)
- Palpation of the temporomandibular joint (TMJ) and examination of the dentition and occlusion
- Observation of the palate for palatal myoclonus
- Fundoscopy may identify the papilledema of benign intracranial hypertension
- Tympanometry for evidence of glue ear, perforation of the tympanic membrane or myoclonic activity
- Pure tone audiometry is essential to document any hearing loss (Figure 7.5)

- Otoacoustic emissions to obtain additional information on cochlear and efferent function
- Auditory brainstem evoked responses may indicate retrocochlear pathology in subjects with asymmetrical tinnitus
- Tinnitus pitch and loudness matching may be performed. Usually the pitch of the tinnitus is found to be at or around the frequency of the maximal hearing loss and the loudness is usually within 15dB of the patient's pure tone threshold at that frequency
- Uncomfortable loudness levels are useful if there is any coexistent hyperacusis
- Medical evaluation in some patients including, full blood count, blood glucose, urea and electrolytes, thyroid function tests and lipids
- MRI is recommended in the presence of asymmetrical tinnitus or hearing loss as 13% of vestibular schwannomas present with asymmetrical tinnitus and normal hearing
- Pulsatile tinnitus may require CT or MR angiography. If the source of tinnitus is not identified on CT or MR angiography and a bruit is heard on auscultation, carotid angiography may be required.

Management

There is a common belief that tinnitus is incurable or untreatable and therefore only a small number of patients (1%) contact physicians or hearing care professionals for help despite its high prevalence. Yet, there are several methods of tinnitus management designed to alleviate the distress associated with tinnitus. Management is best undertaken by a multidisciplinary team comprising an audiovestibular physician or an otolaryngologist, a hearing therapist, an audiologist and a clinical psychologist. Dental treatment

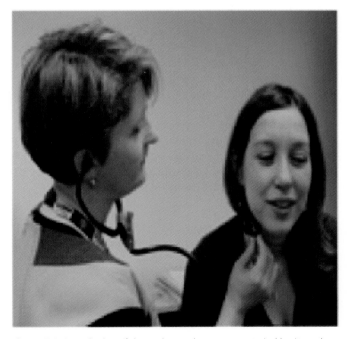

Figure 7.4 Auscultation of the neck may demonstrate cervical bruits and hums arising from cervical arteries or veins.

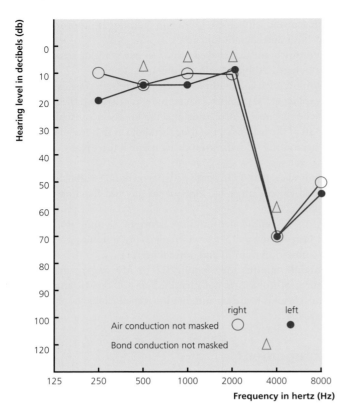

Figure 7.5 Pure tone audiogram showing a sensorineural hearing loss.

or bite realignment can help relieve TMJ pain and associated tinnitus.

Cognitive behavioural therapy

Cognitive behavioural therapy (CBT) is used to identify and alter negative behaviour and thought patterns. The focus of cognitive therapy is on the interpretation that people place upon events rather than the events themselves. If tinnitus per se caused psychological distress, then everyone experiencing tinnitus would experience similar psychological distress, which is clearly untrue. Whereas some patients with tinnitus feel that it indicates the presence of a catastrophic illness, others interpret it as a feature of aging and some patients see their tinnitus in a more positive light. CBT addresses the negative distorted beliefs which surround tinnitus and helps the patient to use structured thinking that results in less anxiety. CBT is believed to be an effective treatment for tinnitus.

Tinnitus retraining therapy (TRT)

Tinnitus retraining therapy (TRT) is designed to help a person retrain the brain to avoid thinking about tinnitus. It uses a combination of counselling together with a non-masking white noise which decreases the contrast between tinnitus and the surrounding environment. Randomised, controlled clinical studies with no treatment and placebo groups are required to ascertain the effectiveness of TRT for the treatment of tinnitus.

Sound therapies

Virtually all sound therapies are combined with some form of counselling. Many tinnitus sufferers get relief from listening to background sounds, such as distant traffic, wind in the trees or waves breaking on the seashore. These sounds can be generated through hearing aids (Figure 7.6) and sound globes. Sound globes (Figure 7.7) are portable devices which sit on the bedside/tabletop and provide a variety of soothing sounds.

Patients with insomnia due to tinnitus may benefit from a pillow speaker (Figures 7.8 and 7.9) or a radio with a time switch. Some sound generators and most compact disc players, mp3 players, etc., can be plugged into a pillow speaker.

Hearing aids

Hearing aids are used increasingly to treat patients with tinnitus. Digital hearing aids seem to alleviate tinnitus more effectively than analogue aids as they can selectively amplify the high frequencies at

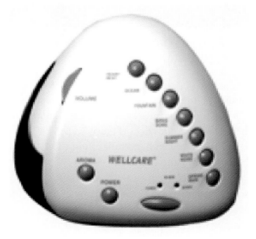

Figure 7.6 Hearing aid. (Source: iStock © Jill Fromer).

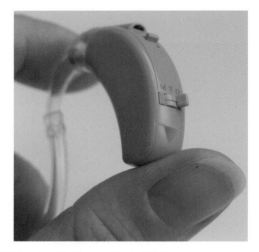

Figure 7.7 Combination aromatherapy and sound relaxation device.

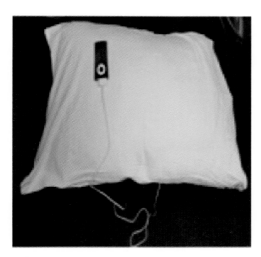

Figure 7.8 Pillow speaker.

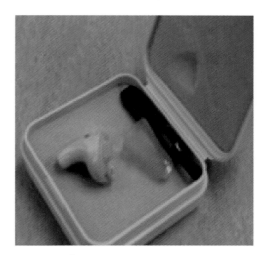

Figure 7.10 Tinnitus white noise generator.

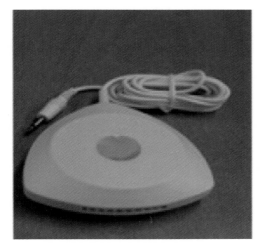

Figure 7.9 Pillow speaker can be attached to an mp3 player.

which tinnitus usually occurs and can also be used for patients with minimal hearing losses, unlike analogue aids.

White noise generators

Masking devices were introduced because patients observed that their tinnitus was more pronounced in quiet surroundings. Current white noise generators are used to obscure rather than obliterate the tinnitus, by producing a gentle rushing sound. The obliteration of tinnitus is seen as being counterproductive in terms of the habituation process, as one cannot habituate to tinnitus which is not audible due to masking. White noise generators are worn behind the ear or in the ear (Figure 7.10). If the patient has a hearing loss as well as tinnitus, the masker and the hearing aid may operate together as one instrument.

Neuromonics

Neuromonics, developed in Australia, combines acoustic stimulation with a structured programme of counselling and support by a clinician skilled in tinnitus rehabilitation. In neuromonics, the audiologist matches the frequency spectrum of the tinnitus to music which overlaps the sound spectrum of the tinnitus. The music stimulates the auditory pathways deprived by hearing loss and engages the limbic system and the autonomic nervous system.

Biofeedback

Biofeedback is a relaxation technique that teaches people to control certain autonomic body functions, such as pulse, muscle tension, and skin temperature. The goal of biofeedback is to help people manage stress, resulting in a reduction in the severity of tinnitus.

Pharmacological treatment

Currently, no pharmacological agent has been shown to cure or consistently alleviate tinnitus. However, some drugs have been shown to be partially effective in some groups of patients (such as zinc in patients with zinc deficiency and selective serotonin re-uptake inhibitors (e.g. Sertraline) in depression). Large clinical trials for promising new treatments are currently underway.

Surgery

Surgery may be indicated in certain otological causes of tinnitus such as vestibular schwannomas, otitis media, perilymph fistulas and otosclerosis.

Further reading

American tinnitus association website. http://www.ata.org.

British tinnitus association website. www.tinnitus.org.uk.

Folmer RL, Griest SE, Meikle MB, Martin WH. Tinnitus severity, loudness, and depression. *Otolaryngol Head Neck Surg* 1999;**121**(1):48–51.

Møller AR, Langguth B, DeRidder D, Kleinjung T. *Textbook of Tinnitus*, Springer, 2010.

Tyler RE. *Tinnitus handbook*, Singular, 2000.

CHAPTER 8

Vertigo and Imbalance

Harold Ludman

King's College Hospital and National Hospital for Neurology and Neurosurgery, London, UK

OVERVIEW

Vertigo is caused by vestibular disturbance and is the result of:

- Intrinsic labyrinthine diseases – Menière's disease, benign paroxysmal positional vertigo and acute vestibular failure
- Spread of disease from an infected middle ear to the labyrinth
- Disease in the brainstem or cerebellum
- General systemic conditions affecting the vestibular system

---

Vertigo, by definition, is an illusion of movement, of the patient or the surroundings. The origin of the name suggests a sense of rotational movement, but should apply to any direction of movement experienced. Imbalance always accompanies vertigo, but is not always due to vertigo and is not a synonym. Imbalance occurs for many reasons without vertigo.

Normal balance needs:

- accurate sensory information from the eyes, proprioceptive receptors and the vestibular labyrinth with coordination of this information within the brain
- normal motor neural control by the central nervous system of an intact musculoskeletal system: normal muscles and joints (Figure 8.1).

Defects in any of these impair balance – with or without vertigo.

Vertigo arises if information from vestibular sources conflicts with data from the other sensory systems, or when a disordered central integration system in the brain does not correctly relate the body's movements to the vestibular input. **Vertigo is always a symptom of vestibular defect.** This may lie in the labyrinth (peripheral) or in its connections within the brain (central). When severe, it is accompanied by nausea and vomiting.

Vertigo is caused by: (a) peripheral vestibular disorders (labyrinthine); (b) middle ear infections spreading to the labyrinth; (c) central vestibular disorders, such as multiple sclerosis, tumours, infarcts; and (d) external damage to the vestibular system – trauma, drugs, anoxia, anaemia, hypoglycaemia, hypotension or viral infections (Box 8.1).

ABC of Ear, Nose and Throat, Sixth Edition.
Edited by Harold Ludman and Patrick J. Bradley.
© 2013 John Wiley & Sons, Ltd. Published 2013 by John Wiley & Sons, Ltd.

Box 8.1 Origins of vertigo

- Peripheral (labyrinthine)
- Central: in the brain (brainstem, cerebellum or higher)

The commonest peripheral vestibular disorders (labyrinthine) are Menière's disease and other forms of endolymphatic hydrops, benign paroxysmal positional vertigo, sudden vestibular failure and vascular disturbances (Box 8.2).

Box 8.2 Peripheral (labyrinthine) disorders

- Menière's disease
- Benign paroxysmal peripheral vertigo (BPPV)
- Sudden vestibular failure

Menière's disease (idiopathic endolymphatic hydrops)

This is a disorder of endolymph control, associated with dilatation of the endolymphatic spaces of the membranous labyrinth (hydrops) (Figure 8.2). This dilatation, or endolymphatic hydrops, may be caused by disorders of the otic capsule, but in Menière's disease it is, by definition, idiopathic.

The disease usually affects only one ear, first producing symptoms between the ages of 30 and 60 years. It is characterised by attacks of violent paroxysmal vertigo, often rotatory, associated with deafness and tinnitus. Attacks occur in clusters with periods of remission, during which balance is normal. Each lasts for several hours, rarely less than 10 minutes or more than 12 hours (Box 8.3), and is accompanied by prostration, nausea and vomiting. A sensation of pressure in the ear, increase or change in the character of tinnitus, pain in the neck or increased deafness often precedes an attack.

Box 8.3 Duration of vertigo

- **Menière's disease**: hours
- **Benign paroxysmal positional vertigo**: seconds only
- **Sudden vestibular failure**: days

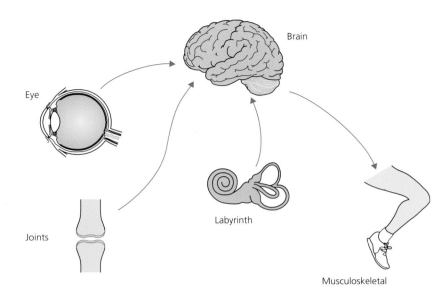

Figure 8.1 Sensory and motor components of balance.

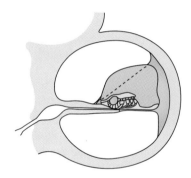

Menière's disease – Dilated scala media in cochlea

Figure 8.2 Menière's disease: dilated scala media in cochlea.

The accompanying deafness is sensorineural and fluctuates noticeably in severity. It is associated with distortion of speech and musical sounds, and with severe discomfort on exposure to loud noise (hyperacusis). Hearing loss may precede the first attack, although both symptoms may first arise together. The vertigo may be so catastrophic that hearing loss is not noticed. Hearing improves during remission, but gradually deteriorates persistently, until its impairment becomes severe. The tinnitus is roaring, low-pitched and worse when hearing is most impaired.

At least 20–30% of patients have disease in both ears. The prevalence of bilateral disease varies widely in reports from different centres, with implications for treatment, and deafness then tends to become more worrying than the vertigo. A variant known as vestibular hydrops produces attacks of episodic vertigo without any auditory symptoms. Another variant of Menière's disease is cochlear hydrops, which is a very common cause of fluctuating hearing loss with tinnitus and distortion, but without vertigo. This common complaint may often be ascribed incorrectly to Eustachian tube obstruction.

Similar vestibular vertigo may be secondary to total cochlear hearing loss from any cause. It has been seen by the author, usually after many years, when the deafness has arisen congenitally, after mumps viral infection or head trauma.

Treatment of Menière's disease

Medical treatment is usually chosen from an armamentarium including histamine agonists such as Betahistine (Serc), often used in the UK as a first choice (but not in the USA, since the FDA consider evidence of efficacy to be insufficient), vasodilator drugs such as nicotinic acid in a dose sufficient to cause flushing, diuretics combined with a sodium-restricted diet and corticosteroids. These treatments may need symptomatic support with antivertigo drugs. This wide range of medication is testimony to our continuing uncertainty about the underlying causes of this disorder.

Operative treatment should be considered if the symptoms are not adequately controlled by medication. Conservative surgical procedures aim to protect hearing, and include decompression of the endolymphatic sac (with or without drainage) and selective division of the vestibular branch of the vestibulocochlear nerve (vestibular neurectomy). Labyrinthectomy, with total destruction of the membranous labyrinth, almost guarantees relief from the vertigo but at the expense of total loss of hearing in that ear. This is often acceptable if the hearing remains only as a painful distorted shred in the affected ear when the other is normal, even though the possible risk of developing disease in the other ear cannot be discounted.

Benign paroxysmal positional vertigo (BPPV)

Benign paroxysmal positional vertigo (BPPV) is the commonest cause of vertigo (Box 8.4). It is provoked by movements of the head (Figure 8.3), usually to one side when turning in bed or on looking upwards. Each attack is violent yet lasts for only a few seconds, and only occurs on assuming the provoking position of the head. There are no auditory symptoms. Episodes usually abate and disappear within a few weeks or months, but they often recur.

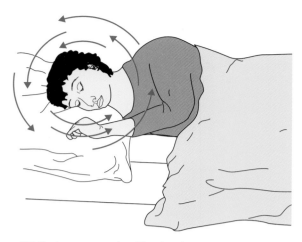

Figure 8.3 Benign paroxysmal positional vertigo.

Box 8.4 Features of BPPV

Features of nystagmus in BPPV on positional testing:

- Rotator beating underlying ear
- Latent period of several seconds before onset
- Abatement after 5–20 s with reduction on repeat testing
- No change in direction while testing

The disorder is caused by detachment of otoconia (calcium carbonate crystals) from the otolith organ of the utricle. They fall into the posterior semicircular canal and distort its cupula when the head is put into the provoking underlying position. Both labyrinths may be affected. Causes may be mechanical in head injury, viral infections or degenerative changes with ageing. Usually there is no recognisable explanation.

Treatment of benign paroxysmal positional vertigo

Most patients need no more than reassurance and avoidance of the provoking head position until recovery. Medication has no useful place. So-called 'repositioning' manoeuvres, involve head movement through a precise sequence of positions designed to force the displaced otoconia out of the posterior canal into the vestibule, and are effective. They are best carried out by experienced people in audiology or neuro-otology units. Some patients may be helped by exercises that deliberately provoke the vertigo, to encourage central compensation for the abnormal vestibular stimuli, but few agree to this unpleasant experience.

Diagnosis is based on eliciting the history of head movement provocation and the brevity of the attacks if the position is maintained. Patients often offer misleading accounts of duration for much longer periods, if they have been repeatedly afflicted over many hours.

Operative measures, which are only used for rare, persistent, severe symptoms, include division of the nerve to the posterior semicircular canal ampulla (singular neurectomy), and obliteration of the lumen of the posterior semicircular canal.

Sudden vestibular failure

Sudden vestibular failure (Figure 8.4) occurs when one peripheral labyrinth suddenly stops working. This may happen for many reasons – head injuries, viral infection, blockage of an end artery supplying the labyrinth, multiple sclerosis, diabetic neuropathy or brainstem encephalitis. It is sometimes confusingly referred to as vestibular neuronitis, or 'labyrinthitis'. These labels are better avoided. The symptoms are sudden vertigo with prostration, nausea and vomiting. There are no auditory features, and the vertigo persists continuously, gradually improving over many days or weeks. Head movements exacerbate vertigo, but after a few days it may cease unless the head is moved. Patients gradually regain balance so that, on the third or fourth day after onset, they may move unsteadily around the room, holding on to objects for support. By the end of 10 days, unsupported walking becomes possible. After 3 weeks gait may seem normal, but patients still feel insecure, particularly in the dark or when tired.

Recovery is slower and less complete in the elderly. It relies on compensating changes within the brain, and imbalance may return temporarily whenever the acquired compensation breaks down, for example through defects in other sensory systems, fatigue, other illnesses, drugs or the cerebral degeneration of old age.

Migraine

Migraine is a common vascular cause of vertigo and may cause symptoms indistinguishable from vertigo. Basilar migraine, affecting teenage girls in the main, is also similar, but may be preceded by posterior cerebral arterial symptoms with disturbance of vision, and may be accompanied by dysarthria and tingling in the hands and feet.

Head injury deserves separate mention. Vertigo often follows concussion and, as mentioned above, BPPV may follow. Perilymph fistula, in which perilymph leaks from the vestibule into the middle ear, may be recognised and treated only by otological referral.

Assessment and diagnosis

The first task is to recognise the symptom as vertigo, and then to determine whether there is any systemic cause or extralabyrinthine

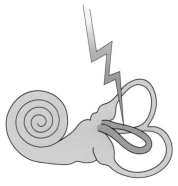

Figure 8.4 Sudden vestibular failure.

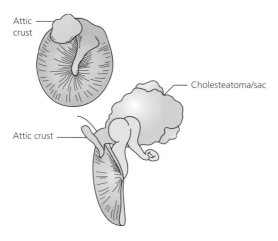

Attic crust

Cholesteatoma/sac

Attic crust

Attic crust may obscure cholesteatoma

Figure 8.5 Attic crust may obscure cholesteatoma.

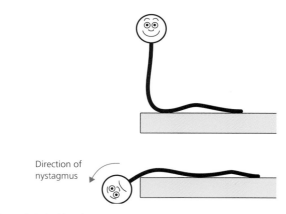

Direction of nystagmus

Figure 8.6 Positional test.

disorder needing urgent investigation – destructive middle ear disease, or any suspicion of central vestibular abnormalities.

The history is especially important to make sure that the complaint is that of a sense of movement. Duration is of paramount importance (Box 8.3), but not easily or reliably attained.

Clinical examination should include assessment of the cardiovascular and central nervous systems. Careful examination of the ears is the only way to recognize destructive middle ear disease by cholesteatoma. Exclusion demands that each tympanic membrane be found to be normal. A waxy crust over the pars flaccida is deceptive, as it may cork the entrance to an attic cholesteatoma (Figure 8.5). If in any doubt, referral for examination with a microscope is essential and anaesthesia may be needed.

Spontaneous jerk nystagmus is always a sign of vestibular disease and is described by the direction of its fast movement. Degree is designated depending on whether it is elicited only with gaze in the direction of the quick beat (1st degree); gazing straight ahead as well (2nd degree); or in all directions (3rd degree). This assessment requires examination of the eyes with good illumination. Inspect in all positions of gaze – but the eyes should not be abducted more than about 30 degrees – until the edge of the iris reaches the caruncle. Certain characteristics of a jerk nystagmus indicate a central cause within the brain. These include: (a) nystagmus persisting for more than a few weeks; (b) change in the direction of beat (defined by its quick component) either with time or change in direction of gaze; (c) beating in directions other than horizontally (e.g. vertically); (d) different jerks in the two eyes (ataxic).

Stance and gait are examined clinically by watching the patient stand on both and then each leg alone with the eyes closed, and while walking heel to toe.

Positional testing

Simple positional testing is the essential diagnostic indicator of BPPV. Seated on a couch, the patient turns the head towards the examiner and is told to keep the eyes open, while watching the examiner's forehead. The tester holds the patient's head, and lays

it rapidly laid backward into a supine position with the head over the edge of the couch at 30° below horizontal (Figure 8.6). The patient is held in that position for at least 30 s, despite protestation, while the eyes are watched for nystagmus. The test is then repeated with the head turned to the other side. Nystagmus provoked by this manoeuvre is always abnormal.

BPPV is always recognisable by this test, but positional testing can also, very rarely, suggest a vestibular lesion somewhere within the posterior cranial fossa. In BPPV, the nystagmus invariably shows the following features: (a) it is rotatory, beating towards the underlying ear; (b) a latent period of some seconds precedes its onset; (c) it abates after 5–20 s held in the provoking position and is less violent on repeated testing; (d) it is accompanied by violent vertigo; (e) it does not change direction during observation. Deviation from even one of these features should suggest a more serious central cause requiring further investigation, preferably by MRI scan.

Neuro-otological investigations of vestibular function – Many tests are available for full assessment. They start with detailed assessment of **auditory** function, by pure tone audiometry in a soundproofed room (Figure 8.7), and include recording of brainstem evoked

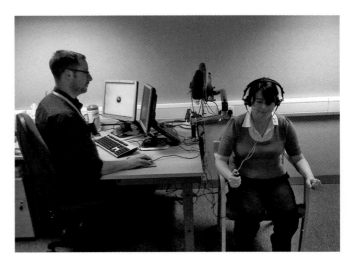

Figure 8.7 Audiometry in sound proofed booth.

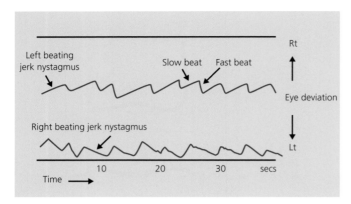

Figure 8.8 Caloric induced nystagmus. The upward beats show the fast components of the jerk nystagmus.

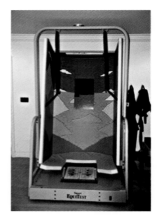

Figure 8.9 Posturography equipment.

responses to auditory stimuli, which are valuable for recognising retrocochlear hearing losses that may be caused by vestibular schwannomas (acoustic neuromas).

Vestibular function is assessed by many tests including the Fitzgerald–Hallpike caloric test, in which each lateral semicircular canal is vicariously stimulated by irrigation of the ears with water at temperatures above and below body temperature (30 and 44°C). Ice-cold water may be used for an apparently 'dead' labyrinth. Rotation tests, when the whole body is turned in a specially designed chair, at variable angular acceleration induce nystagmus, which is recorded by electronystagmography (Figure 8.8). These proffer valuable diagnostic information about both spontaneous and induced nystagmus (Box 8.5). Posturography (Figure 8.9) offers ways to assess body position under different external stimuli.

Box 8.5 **Features of central nystagmus**

Central *spontaneous* nystagmus is indicated by:

- Persistence for several weeks
- Change in direction (of quick component) with time or direction of gaze
- Direction other than horizontal
- Ataxic beating

Symptomatic treatment of vertigo

Symptoms may be relieved by sedatives such as prochlorperazine, cinnarizine and other antihistamines. Diazepam is also useful. In a severe attack such as after vestibular failure, bedrest will be necessary whatever the cause. Drugs may be given intramuscularly or as suppositories. Once the acute stage is over, sedatives are continued in small doses for several weeks or months.

If vestibular deficit – rather than irritation of a labyrinthine system – is pronounced, vestibular sedatives may exacerbate the symptoms. This often happens in the degenerative changes of old age, in bilateral Menière's disease or after ototoxic drug damage. Graded head and eye movement exercises, designed to accelerate the process of central compensation, can help patients. These "head exercises" should be taught and supervised by specially trained physiotherapists.

Other treatment is directed at identified causes, including surgical exploration of any middle ear in which cholesteatomatous erosion of the middle ear is suspected.

Further reading

Ludman H, Wright T (eds) *Diseases of the Ear*, 6th edn. Arnold-Hodder, London, 1998.

Luxon LM (ed.) *Textbook of Audiological Medicine*. Taylor & Francis, London, 2003.

http://www.menieres.org.uk/

CHAPTER 9

Facial Palsy

Iain Swan

Glasgow Royal Infirmary, Glasgow, UK

OVERVIEW

- Facial weakness or paralysis must always be investigated
- Important causes to exclude are:
  - Middle ear disease: urgent treatment is necessary
  - Parotid malignancy
- Idiopathic or 'Bell's palsy' is the most common diagnosis but this can be suggested *only* when any other causes have been excluded
- The most effective treatment for Bell's palsy is corticosteroids in the first 72 hours. Current evidence suggests that other treatments are ineffective
- Patients with herpes zoster oticus present with severe pain as well as facial weakness
- Other causes of facial palsy are uncommon but must be considered if the palsy progresses or does not improve

---

Definition

A facial palsy is weakness of the muscles of facial expression, from disease of the VIIth cranial nerve, or from disease in adjacent structures.

Anatomy

The facial nerve leaves the facial nucleus, in the brainstem, and passes through the internal auditory meatus beside the VIIIth cranial nerve. After the geniculate ganglion, it runs horizontally across the middle ear in the fallopian canal, just above the oval window, then turns vertically downward, where it supplies the stapedius muscle before leaving the temporal bone through the stylomastoid foramen. It enters the parotid gland where it divides into five main branches distributed to the muscles of facial expression. In the middle ear it also contains secretomotor fibres to the submandibular and sublingual salivary glands and taste fibres from the anterior two-thirds of the tongue, via the chorda tympani.

ABC of Ear, Nose and Throat, Sixth Edition.
Edited by Harold Ludman and Patrick J. Bradley.
© 2013 John Wiley & Sons, Ltd. Published 2013 by John Wiley & Sons, Ltd.

Presentation

Patients present with weakness of the muscles of facial expression (Figure 9.1). The affected side of the face droops and they may be unable to close their eye. They may complain of hyperacusis due to paralysis of the stapedius muscle in the midde ear. In severe cases, there may be a metallic taste due to a change of taste sensation on one side of the tongue. Reduced lacrimation causes dryness of the affected eye. Poor mouth closure can cause drooling and difficulty with eating.

The great majority of facial palsies are from lower motor neurone lesions. Upper motor neurone lesions arise from disease, such as strokes, in the brain. In upper motor neurone lesions, the patient can still move the upper part of the face (i.e. the forehead), because of crossover pathways in the brainstem, but the distinction may be difficult.

Clinical testing can sometimes help to localise the area of damage to the nerve. Schirmer's test can be used to test lacrimation. A small strip of filter paper is hung from the lower eyelids and the flow of fluid compared. Normal lacrimation would suggest that the lesion is distal to the geniculate ganglion. Testing taste sensation on the anterior two-thirds of the tongue would indicate whether the chorda tympani was affected. The stapedius reflex can be measured. These tests are of limited value as they have poor correlation with the site of damage, and have been superseded by MRI when localisation is required.

Aetiology

Most facial palsies (nearly 75%) are of unknown origin (i.e. idiopathic), so-called 'Bell's palsy'. Aetiologies are listed in Table 9.1.

Bell's palsy

Bell's palsy is an idiopathic, lower motor neurone facial palsy. The onset is over a few hours, commonly arising overnight. Patients often complain of an aching pain around the ear, often preceding the onset of the palsy. Severe otalgia suggests herpes zoster (see below). Patients may also complain of facial numbness, hyperacusis and altered taste. There is an annual incidence of 20–30 cases per 100 000 of the population. Individuals can be affected at any age, but young and middle-aged adults are the most likely to be affected.

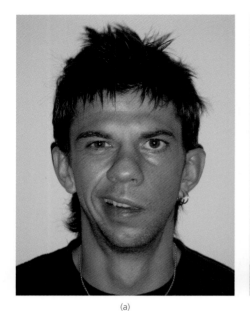

(a)

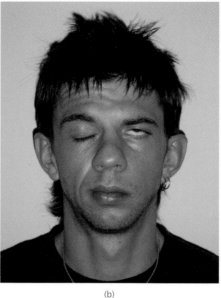

(b)

Figure 9.1 A left-sided lower motor neurone facial nerve palsy: (a) note generalized muscle weakness of left side of the face – forehead, cheek and mouth; (b) a positive Bell's phenomenon when attempting to close the left eye.

Table 9.1 Aetiologies of facial palsy.

Lower motor neurone facial palsy
Idiopathic	Bell's palsy
Infection	Acute otitis media
	Chronic otitis media, especially cholesteatoma
	Herpes zoster (Ramsay Hunt Syndrome)
	Lyme disease
Neoplasm	Malignant parotid neoplasms
	Middle ear carcinoma
	Facial neuroma
Trauma	
Other	Sarcoidosis
	Wegener's granulomatosis
	Multiple sclerosis
	Melkersson–Rosenthal syndrome

Upper motor neurone facial palsy
CVAs
Intracranial tumours

Table 9.2 House–Brackmann 1985 grading of facial palsy.

Grade	Definition
I	Normal symmetrical function in all areas
II	Slight weakness noticeable only on close inspection
	Complete eye closure with minimal effort
	Slight asymmetry of smile with maximal effort
	Synkinesis barely noticeable, contracture, or spasm absent
III	Obvious weakness, but not disfiguring
	May not be able to lift eyebrow
	Complete eye closure and strong but asymmetrical mouth movement with maximal effort
	Obvious, but not disfiguring synkinesis, mass movement or spasm
IV	Obvious disfiguring weakness
	Inability to lift brow
	Incomplete eye closure and asymmetry of mouth with maximal effort
	Severe synkinesis, mass movement, spasm
V	Motion barely perceptible
	Incomplete eye closure, slight movement corner mouth
	Synkinesis, contracture, and spasm usually absent
VI	No movement, loss of tone, no synkinesis, contracture, or spasm

Pregnant women and individuals with diabetes are thought to be at greater risk.

Aetiology

The symptoms of Bell's palsy probably arise from inflammation or swelling of the facial nerve, but where precisely is uncertain. The cause is unclear. Herpes simplex virus (HSV) has been postulated but no good evidence has been found. Inflammatory and immunological causes have also been suggested.

Diagnosis

Bell's palsy is a diagnosis of exclusion. The ears and the parotid gland must be carefully examined to exclude middle ear disease and parotid neoplasms. A brief neurological examination should exclude other neurological conditions. The degree of the palsy should be recorded, most commonly by using the House–Brackmann grading system (Table 9.2). This is clinically useful as it provides a baseline measurement which allows assessment of the patient's progress. With a good clinical history and examination, investigations are unhelpful.

Electrophysiological tests can be used – electroneuronography and electromyography. These give no useful information in incomplete paralysis where there is a high chance of good recovery. They may be of some help in complete paralysis when surgical decompression is being considered. Degeneration of more than 90% suggests poor recovery. Surgery is sometimes considered in these cases although the evidence is lacking.

Treatment

The most important part of initial treatment is advising the patient of the need to protect the affected eye. It may become dry, particularly at night, and eye closure may be incomplete. Damage to the cornea may result. Treatment includes artificial tears and an eye patch or other protective measures, particularly at night and when out of doors on a windy day.

There have been many trials of treatment for Bell's palsy but the results were, for many years, inconclusive. However, in more recent years there have been several large, high-quality trials of treatment and Cochrane Reviews of these trials have been published. These have shown that patients treated in the first 72 h with corticosteroids have a significantly better chance of complete recovery. Prednisolone is the most commonly used corticosteroid in a dosage of 1mg/kg for 7 days. Treatment with antiviral agents alone is no more effective than placebo and is worse than corticosteroids. Treatment with antivirals and corticosteroids is no better than corticosteroids alone. Other treatments such as acupuncture and physiotherapy have not been shown to be effective. Surgical decompression is considered in some severe cases but there is no good evidence that it is effective.

If there is no recovery of facial function, after many months surgical procedures may reduce disability. Eye closure can be improved by gold weights in the upper lid and canthal slings to elevate the lower lid. Fascial slings can elevate the corner of the mouth. Cross-facial anastomoses can provide reinnervation to the paralysed facial muscles. Occasionally anastomosis of the facial nerve with the hypoglossal nerve can be of some help.

Prognosis

In the majority of cases (70–75%) there is complete recovery of facial function, with partial recovery in a further 10–15%. Most patients with Bell's palsy begin to notice improvement in their palsy within 2–3 weeks of the onset of symptoms, though recovery in some patients may be in 3–6 months. The prognosis is better in incomplete palsy (about 95% complete recovery), when improvement is early and in younger patients. A small number of patients (3–7%) suffer recurrence of the palsy years later. No further recovery is likely after 6 months without improvement.

In some cases, particularly severe ones, when there is some recovery the patient will experience facial synkinesis. They experience involuntary muscle movement accompanying voluntary movement, for example smiling induces contraction of the eye muscles.

If there is no evidence of recovery within 3–4 months, a diagnosis of Bell's palsy must be reconsidered.

Herpes zoster oticus (Ramsay Hunt syndrome)

Ramsay Hunt syndrome is an acute unilateral facial palsy caused by reactivation of varicella zoster virus (VZV) in the geniculate ganglion. It is more common in the immunosuppressed and in the elderly. Patients present with moderate to severe pain around the ear, often with few signs at this stage (Figure 9.2). They develop

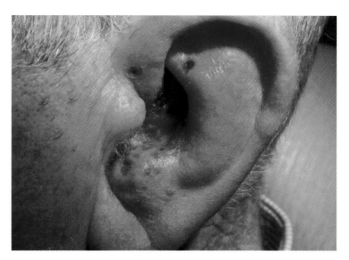

Figure 9.2 View of left pinna showing a diffuse weeping rash around the conchal bowel and the external auditory canal.

a facial palsy, often accompanied by audiovestibular symptoms of hearing loss, tinnitus and vertigo. They usually also notice loss of taste on the anterior two thirds of the tongue. Vesicles often appear 2–3 days later in the concha and sometimes on the ipsilateral anterior two-thirds of the tongue.

Many patients, 30–50%, do not recover full facial function. The facial palsy is commonly more severe than in Bell's palsy. Only 10% of cases with complete facial palsy recover fully if untreated. Early treatment with high dose antivirals (e.g. valcyclovir) and corticosteroids (e.g. prednisolone 1mg/kg/day for 7 days) is widely recommended. However, there is no evidence that they are effective.

Otitis media

Facial palsy is a rare complication of otitis media. Mild weakness may occur in acute otitis media, thought to be due to congenital dehiscence of the facial nerve in the middle ear. This recovers quickly and does not influence the treatment of the otitis media.

In chronic otitis media (COM), facial palsy occurs more commonly in erosive active squamous COM (cholesteatoma) (Figure 9.3) but can also occur in mucosal COM. It is usually associated with dehiscence of the facial nerve in the fallopian canal and granulation tissue overlying the nerve. In the presence of facial nerve palsy, active chronic otitis media should be managed urgently and almost always surgically. Complete recovery of facial function can be expected in most cases after early, careful surgical management.

Lyme disease

Lyme disease is a rare cause of facial palsy. The cause is infection with a spirochete, *Borrelia burgdorferi*, which is transmitted by tick bite in endemic areas of the world. There is a flu-like illness, often with a rash. Cranial neuropathies can occur several weeks later in untreated cases. Facial palsy is the commonest and is bilateral in 75% of cases. Treatment is with antibiotics (doxycycline or amoxicillin for 14–21 days) and full recovery is likely.

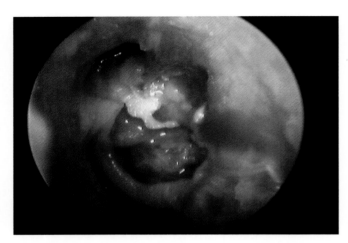

Figure 9.3 View of the right tympanic membrane area with a large central perforation, ossicular erosion and an attic defect all caused by cholesteatoma.

Malignant otitis externa

Malignant otitis externa is an uncommon infective condition, most commonly affecting elderly diabetic patients (see Chapter 2). Facial palsy can occur in advanced cases.

Neoplasms

Malignant neoplasms of the parotid gland and the middle ear are rare causes of facial palsy. They should be excluded by clinical examination. Facial neuromas are uncommon. It should be suspected in cases of apparently idiopathic facial palsy which do not recover or continue to progress. It is not a diagnosis which needs to be considered in the early stages of facial palsy as surgical treatment will usually result in a total facial palsy, and for this reason is not considered urgent.

Trauma

Facial palsy can occur after head injury with fracture of the temporal bone. Delayed onset palsy, a few hours after injury, is due to swelling around the nerve. Treatment with corticosteroids is recommended and a good recovery is likely. Immediate onset palsy may be caused by the nerve being trapped in a fracture line, or torn. Surgical exploration should be considered, but the patient's general condition usually precludes this. High-density imaging is necessary to diagnose the type and site of injury. Many immediate onset facial palsies recover with conservative management.

Other causes

Facial palsy can occur in sarcoidosis but is a very rare presenting sign. It can also occur in Wegener's granulomatosis secondary to middle ear involvement. Multiple sclerosis can cause a facial palsy which can be intermittent; as with other neurological causes, there are usually other signs. Melkersson–Rosenthal syndrome can cause recurrent facial palsy, often contralateral. There may be a fissured tongue and a positive family history is common. It may rarely arise in children with hypertension.

Further reading

Adour KK, Wingerd J. Idiopathic facial paralysis (Bell's palsy): factors affecting severity and outcome in 446 patients. *Neurology* 1974;**24**:112–16.

Gilden DH. Clinical practice. Bell's Palsy. *New Engl J Med* 2004;**351**(13): 1323–31.

House JW, Brackmann DE. Facial nerve grading system. *Otolaryngol Head Neck Surg* 1985;**93**:146–7.

Lockhart P, Daly F, Pitkethly M, Comerford N, Sullivan F. Antiviral treatment for Bell's palsy (idiopathic facial paralysis). *Cochrane Database Syst Rev* 2009;Issue 4:CD001869.

McAllister K, Walker D, Donnan PT, Swan I. Surgical interventions for the early management of Bell's palsy. *Cochrane Database Syst Rev* 2011;Issue 2: CD007468.

Salinas RA, Alvarez G, Daly F, Ferreira J. Corticosteroids for Bell's palsy (idiopathic facial paralysis). *Cochrane Database Syst Rev* 2010;Issue 3:CD001942.

Uscategui T, Doree C, Chamberlain IJ, Burton MJ. Antiviral therapy for Ramsay Hunt syndrome (herpes zoster oticus with facial palsy) in adults. *Cochrane Database Syst Rev* 2008;Issue 4:CD006851. Review.

CHAPTER 10

Facial Pain

Lisha McLelland and Nick S. Jones

Nottingham University Hospitals, Queen's Medical Centre Campus, Nottingham, UK

OVERVIEW

- A careful history is essential for an accurate diagnosis
- In the absence of any nasal symptoms or signs, facial pain is unlikely to be due to sinus disease
- Patients with a normal CT scan are unlikely to have pain due to rhinosinusitis (NB CT changes on their own are not diagnostic of rhinosinusitis)
- If it is not possible to make a diagnosis at the first consultation, it is helpful to ask the patient to keep a diary of their symptoms, carry out a trial of medical treatment and review
- If a patient has facial pain as well as nasal obstruction and a loss of sense of smell, which is worse with the common cold or flying, then he or she is likely to be helped by nasal medical or, if that fails, surgical treatment
- Patients with purulent secretions and facial pain are likely to benefit from treatment directed at rhinosinusitis

---

In patients with facial pain it is important to get the diagnosis right in order to prevent the unnecessary prescription of medication or surgery. Most people are aware that the sinuses lie behind the facial bones; therefore, it is not surprising that many believe that the cause of their facial pain is their sinuses. However, rhinosinusitis is often not the cause of facial pain.

A structured approach is essential; this can be aided by using an anatomical or pathological surgical sieve. An anatomical approach would focus the history on the site of pain, for example nose, sinus, teeth, temporomandibular joint or eyes. An alternative would be a pathological sieve, for example see Table 10.1.

A combination of both approaches gives the seven key catagories of facial pain; rhinological pain, dental pain, vascular pain, neruralgias, midfacial pain, atypical facial pain and pain secondary to neoplasia. A careful history is essential for correct diagnosis.

Eight questions form the basis of an algorithm that will help towards a diagnosis.

1 **Where is the pain?** Ask the patient to point to the site of the pain, this locates the pain and the gesture often provides information about its nature and its emotional significance to the patient.

ABC of Ear, Nose and Throat, Sixth Edition.
Edited by Harold Ludman and Patrick J. Bradley.
© 2013 John Wiley & Sons, Ltd. Published 2013 by John Wiley & Sons, Ltd.

Table 10.1 Pathological surgical sieve.

	Example
Infection	Dental abscess, acute rhinosinusitis
Inflammation	Acute rhinosinusitis
Trauma	Fractured nose
Tumour	Intracranial tumours
Vascular	Migraine
Neurological	Trigeminal autonomic cephalgia, trigeminal neuralgia, tension-type headache, midfacial segment pain
Iatrogenic	Surgery
Idiopathic	Atypical facial pain

2 **Does it radiate?** Pain extending either across the midline or across neurological dermatomes is less likely to have a physical basis.

3 **What is the character of the pain?** A sensation of pressure is in keeping with tension-type headache or midfacial segment pain. Patients with migraine report a throbbing pain and a burning or gnawing pain is characteristic of neuropathic pain.

4 **How long or frequent is each episode?** Is the pain continuous or intermittent? Is it present daily, is there a pattern or is it progressive? A common misconception is that migraine only lasts a few hours, but it can last up to 72 hours. Symmetrical pain persisting over weeks in the cheeks, behind the eyes, the bridge of the nose or affecting the forehead is more likely to be due to midfacial segment pain rather than rhinosinusitis. The periodicity of symptoms may be a pointer to the diagnosis. For example, being woken in the morning by very severe facial pain that lasts less than 1 hour suggests cluster headache. A progressive headache associated with nausea or effortless vomiting means that an intracranial lesion should be excluded.

5 **What precipitates the pain?** Unilateral pain following a cold and associated with nasal obstruction and a persistent nasal discharge is indicative of infective rhinosinusitis.

6 **What relieves the pain?** What treatments have been tried and what was the effect. Tension-type headache does not respond to analgesics, whereas patients with migraine often report that lying quietly in a dark room helps.

7 **Are there any associated symptoms?** Nausea accompanying the pain is characteristic, although not diagnostic, of migraine. Ipsilateral lacrimation, rhinorrhoea or nasal obstruction can occur with trigeminal autonomic cephalgias.

8 What effect does it have on daily life and sleep? Should the patient describe marked unrelenting pain, yet have a normal sleep pattern, atypical facial pain should be considered in the differential diagnosis.

Facial pain often has some emotional significance. For some patients, facial pain may be greatly affected by emotional distress, anxiety or the psychological harm the patient associates with disease, trauma or surgery. It may sometimes be the means by which they obtain secondary gain. The presence of marked psychological overlay does not mean that there is no underlying organic problem, but it is a relative contraindication to surgical treatment. If there is a big discrepancy between the patient's affect and the description of the pain, the organic component of the illness may be of relatively minor importance. Should the diagnosis be elusive, re-taking the history at a further consultation may be helpful, as well as asking the patient to keep a symptom diary.

Examination

This should include anterior rhinoscopy as well as endoscopic assessment of the nasal cavity, sinus ostia and postnasal space. This is frequently normal. Examination of the eyes, ears, oral cavity and face should be included as indicated from the history.

Investigations

Incidental radiological findings are common and limit the usefulness of computed tomography (CT) and magnetic resonance imaging (MRI) in the diagnosis of facial pain. Note that a third of asymptomatic patients have incidental mucosal changes on CT, and so radiographic changes are not diagnostic of rhinosinusitis. If they are performed, any positive findings should be interpreted with caution in the light of the history and endoscopic findings.

Making the diagnosis

Infection

Nose and sinus infection
Acute sinusitis usually follows an acute upper respiratory tract infection. Pain is usually unilateral, intense, associated with fever and unilateral nasal obstruction, and there may be a purulent discharge. Chronic sinusitis is often painless, causing nasal obstruction due to mucosal hypertrophy, and with a purulent discharge that continues throughout the day. An acute exacerbation can cause pain, but this rarely lasts for more than a few days. The pain is often a unilateral dull ache around the medial canthus of the eye, although more severe facial pain can occur, and in maxillary sinusitis toothache often occurs. An increase in the severity of pain on bending forward is traditionally thought to be diagnostic of sinusitis, but in fact many types of facial pain and headache are made worse by this action. The key points in the history of sinogenic pain are an association with rhinological symptoms and a response to medical treatment. Facial swelling is uncommon and usually due to other pathology such as dental sepsis. Nasendoscopy is very helpful, if not essential, in making or excluding the diagnosis of sinusitis. A normal nasal cavity, showing no evidence of middle meatal mucopus or inflammatory changes, makes a diagnosis of sinogenic pain most unlikely. Patients who report intermittent symptoms of facial pain can be asked to return for endoscopic examination when they are symptomatic. In patients with genuine sinusitis, over 75% have been shown to have their facial pain alleviated by endoscopic sinus surgery.

Dental Infection
Dental infection is a recognised cause of facial pain and swelling. However, there is usually clinical evidence of pain as the tooth is painful on percussion or there is inflammation of the surrounding gingiva.

Eye Infection
Orbital pain can also be caused by uveitis, keratitis and glaucoma. Disease involving the optic nerve results in reduced acuity and colour vision.

Inflammation
Nose and sinus
Facial pain without any nasal symptoms is unlikely to be due to sinusitis. Transient facial pain in patients with other symptoms and signs of rhinosinusitis can occur with pressure changes when flying, diving or skiing, but this resolves as the pressure within the sinuses equalizes through perfusion with the surrounding vasculature. The evidence that a vacuum within a blocked sinus can cause protracted pain is poor.

The theories that implicate contact points as a cause of facial pain have been questioned, as the prevalence of contact points has been found to be the same in an asymptomatic population as in a symptomatic population, and when they were present in symptomatic patients with unilateral pain, they were present in the contralateral side to the pain in 50% of these patients. Nowhere else in the body does mucosa–mucosa contact cause pain. Anatomical variations within the nose/sinuses have been said to be responsible for causing pain, but case-controlled studies have shown that these variations are as common in a symptomatic as an asymptomatic population.

Dental pain
Pain originating from the dental pulp may be poorly localised and radiate. Dentino-enamel defects often give a sharp localised pain. All too often pain in the upper jaw is thought to be of dental or sinus origin, and it may not be until several extractions or sinus surgical procedures have been performed without benefit that it becomes apparent that the pain was and is neurological and is often due to 'phantom tooth pain'. It is important not to perform surgery or extract teeth without good objective evidence that they are the cause.

Temporomandibular joint pain
Temporomandibular joint dysfunction is most commonly unilateral (90%) and usually occurs in young adults with a history of bruxism, clenching, trauma, recent dental work, anxiety, enthusiastic

kissing or cradling the telephone between the jaw and the shoulder. Pain is caused by pterygoid spasm and is described as a deep, dull ache that may masquerade as toothache or earache. There is often a superimposed sharper component that may radiate down the jaw or over the side of the face or temple. Clicking of the temporomandibular joint is an unreliable sign, whereas trismus and deviation of the jaw from the midline on opening help confirm the diagnosis; there may be tenderness of the joint on palpation.

Eye-related pain

Uncorrected optical refractive errors can cause headaches, but their importance is exaggerated. Pain on ocular movement is suggestive of optic neuritis or scleritis. It is vital to recognise acute glaucoma that may cause severe orbital pain and headache. The patient may see haloes around lights, and may feel very unwell with vomiting. Testing visual acuity is important in assessing intraocular disease and, if it is abnormal with the patient's glasses (if they are used), an ophthalmological opinion is needed.

Trauma

Post traumatic or surgical pain

Occasionally pain can persist following a nasal fracture or following nasal surgery. It is possible that peripheral regenerative or deafferent changes may influence the sensory nuclear complex of the trigeminal brainstem causing neuropathic pain. However, the psychological effects of assault, ongoing litigation or dissatisfaction following surgery may affect pain perception.

Tumour

It is rare for tumours involving the head and face to present with pain. Where pain is a symptom it tends to be progressive in nature, often associated with suspicious symptoms or focal neurology. Malignant lesions of the nose and sinus such as carcinoma and melanoma may remain relatively asymptomatic until a late stage.

Neurovascular

Trigeminal autonomic cephalgias

Cluster headache

Cluster headache typically presents with a very severe unilateral stabbing or burning pain, which may be frontal, temporal, ocular, or over the cheek (Figure 10.1). There may be associated ipsilateral symptoms such as rhinorrhoea, nasal obstruction, lacrimation or conjunctival injection and signs, for example myosis, eyelid oedema, facial flushing and sweating may be seen. It is most common in men aged between 30 and 50 years. The patient is awakened in the early hours, often walking around the bedroom in distress, with the pain lasting between 30 min and 2 h. It may be precipitated by alcohol intake.

Chronic paroxysmal hemicrania

Chronic paroxysmal hemicrania is an excruciating pain occurring in women at any time of the night or day. It can affect the frontal, orbital, cheek or temporal regions and lasts around 30 min. The patient can experience multiple episodes in 24 h and ipsilateral

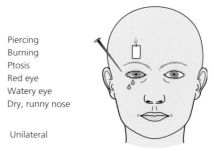

Piercing
Burning
Ptosis
Red eye
Watery eye
Dry, runny nose

Unilateral

Figure 10.1 The features of cluster headache.

symptoms such as rhinorrhoea, nasal obstruction, lacrimation or conjunctival injection and signs for example myosis, eyelid oedema, facial flushing and sweating may be seen, as with cluster headaches. Response to Indomethacin is needed to make the diagnosis.

SUNCT (short-lasting unilateral neuralgiform headache attacks with conjunctival injection and tearing)

SUNCT is a syndrome with frequent short episodes of unilateral facial pain lasting from seconds to minutes associated with ipsilateral lacrimation and conjunctival injection.

Migraine

Migraine causes severe headache, but in a small proportion of patients it can affect the cheek, orbit and forehead. It is described as sharp, severe and throbbing pain that lasts up to 72 h. It may occur with or without aura. There is good evidence for the role of vascular change in migraine with aura (spreading oligaemia); however, there is increasing support for the role of neurotransmitters, peripheral nerve terminals and potentiation within the central nervous system in migraine without aura. Migraine is invariably accompanied by nausea and may be associated with photophobia and phonophobia. Premenstruation, diet, stress or stress withdrawal can induce an attack, as with classical migraine. There is often a family history of migraine. Treatment with triptans is affective during acute attacks. Pizotifen or beta-blockers may be used for prophylaxis.

Neurological

Tension-type headache

The precise biomechanics of tension-type headaches are not understood but peripheral and central pain mechanisms are thought to be central. Tension-type headache has the qualities of non-pulsatile tightness or pressure. It usually affects the forehead, temple and often the suboccipital area as well (Figure 10.2). It may be episodic or chronic (>15 days per month, >3 months), and is only occasionally helped by non-steroidal anti-inflammatory drugs. Typically, patients take large quantities of analgesics yet say that they produce little benefit. Hyperaesthesia of the skin or muscles of the forehead often occurs and tenderness to palpation over the pericranium. The majority of patients with this condition respond to low-dose amitriptyline, but it takes 6–8 weeks to work and they then require treatment for 6 months. It is sensible to inform patients that amitriptyline is also used in higher doses for other conditions such

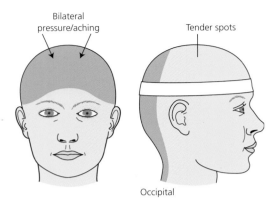

Figure 10.2 Diagramatic representation of the features of tension-type headache.

as depression. If amitriptyline fails, then relief may be obtained from gabapentin or pregabalin.

Midfacial segment pain

Midfacial segment pain causes a symmetrical sensation of pressure or tightness across the middle third of the face, and it is not uncommon to have coexisting tension-type headache. Some patients may say that the nose feels blocked, although they will have no nasal airway obstruction. The areas of pressure involve the bridge of the nose, either side of the nose, the peri-orbital or retro-orbital regions, or across the cheeks (Figure 10.3). The pain lasts for hours or can be continuous. There may be hyperaesthesia of the skin and soft tissues over the affected area on examination, and gently touching the affected area is enough to cause discomfort. Sometimes the patient says that their face is swollen yet there is no evidence of swelling or underlying bony disease. Nasal endoscopy is normal as is CT of the paranasal sinuses. There is no consistent exacerbating

or relieving factor. Therefore, midfacial segment pain has all the characteristics of tension-type headache, with the exception that it affects the midface. The majority of patients with this condition respond to low-dose amitriptyline and are treated in the same way as patients with tension-type headache. It seems likely that the underlying pathology in midfacial segment pain is similar to that in tension-type headache. It is of interest that, if surgery is mistakenly performed as a treatment for midfacial segment pain, the pain may sometimes abate temporarily, only to return after several weeks to months.

Trigeminal neuralgia

Trigeminal neuralgia is more common in women over 40 years of age, with a peak incidence between 50 and 60 years. Patients complain of paroxysms of agonizing, lancinating pain induced by a specific trigger point, although there is a refractory period of more than 30 s. In more than a third of sufferers, the pain occurs in both the maxillary and mandibular divisions, whilst in a fifth it is confined to the mandibular region and in 3% to the ophthalmic division. Typical trigger sites are the lips and the nasolabial folds, but pain may also be triggered by touching the gingivae. Remissions are common but it is not unusual for the attacks to increase in frequency and severity. Treatment is with carbamazepine or gabapentin. In refractory cases, microvascular decompression or stereotactic radiosurgery may be considered. In patients under 40 years old, it is most commonly due to disseminating sclerosis and a MRI scan is recommended.

Postherpetic neuralgia

Pain following herpes zoster infection may occur in up to 50% of elderly patients with shingles. Recovery may take months. Treatment with antiviral drugs during an acute attack may reduce

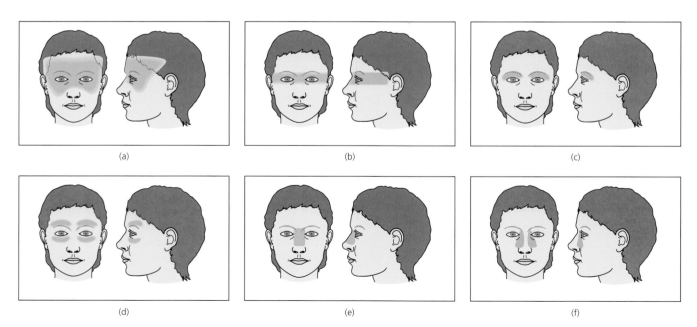

(a) (b) (c)

(d) (e) (f)

Figure 10.3 (a)–(f) Distribution of the symmetrical symptoms of pressure in midfacial segment pain.

symptoms and it helps to get the pain under control early in its evolution.

Idiopathic

Atypical facial pain is a diagnosis that should only be made reluctantly and it is important to exclude organic disease. The history is often vague or inconsistent with widespread pain extending from the face to other areas of the head and neck. Pain is typically deep and ill-defined, changes location, is unexplainable on an anatomical basis, occurs almost daily and is sometimes fluctuating, sometimes continuous, has no precipitating factors and is not relieved by analgesics. Specific questioning about the symptoms often results in vague answers. The pain does not wake the patient up, and although the patient reports that they cannot sleep, they will often look well rested. It is more common in women over the age of 40. There may be a history of other pain syndromes and the patient's extensive records show minimal progress despite various medications. Many patients with atypical facial pain exhibit evidence of psychological disturbance or a history of depression and are unable to function normally as a result of their pain. The management of such patients is challenging and confrontation is nearly always counterproductive. A good starting point is to reassure the patients that you recognise that they have genuine pain, and an empathetic consultation with an explanation should be conducted. Drug treatment revolves around a gradual build-up to the higher analgesic and antidepressant levels of amitriptyline (75–100 mg) at night.

Conclusions

The majority of patients who present with facial pain and headaches believe they have 'sinus trouble'. There is an increasing awareness amongst otorhinolaryngologists that neurological causes are responsible for a large proportion of headache and facial pain. We believe that patients with facial pain who have no objective evidence of sinus disease (endoscopy negative) are unlikely to be helped by nasal medical or surgical treatment. In these patients, other diagnoses should be considered and appropriate medical treatment tried. A comprehensive examination including nasendoscopy is highly desirable in order to confirm or refute the diagnosis of sinusitis. Any association between anatomical findings such as a concha bullosa or a septal deviation and facial pain has been discredited and surgery should be avoided for these incidental variations.

Further reading

Abu-Bakra M, Jones NS. The prevalence of nasal contact points in a population with facial pain and a control population. *J Laryngol Otol* 2001;**115**:629–32.

Daudia A, Jones NS. Facial migraine in a rhinological setting. *Clin Otolaryngol* 2002;**27**:521–5.

Hughes R, Jones NS. The role of endoscopy in outpatient management. *Clin Otolaryngol* 1998;**23**:224–6.

Jensen R, Olesen J. Tension-type headache: an update on mechanisms and treatment. *Curr Opin Neurol* 2000;**13**:285–9.

Jones NS. Midfacial segment pain: implications for rhinitis and sinusitis. Curr Allergy Asthma Rep 2004;**4**:187–92.

Khan O, Majumdar S, Jones NS. Facial pain after sinus surgery and trauma. *Clin Otolaryngol* 2002;**27**:171–4.

Marshall A, Jones NS. The utility of radiological studies in the diagnosis and management of rhinosinusitis. *Curr Infect Dis Rep* 2003;**5**:199–204.

Scully C, Felix DH. Oral Medicine: orofacial pain. *Br Dental J* 2006;**200**:75–80.

Renton T. An update on pain. *Br Dental J* 2008;**204**:335–8.

Sessle BJ. Acute and chronic craniofacial pain: brainstem mechanisms of nociceptive transmission and neuroplasticity, and other clinical correlates. *Crit Rev Oral Biol Med* 2000;**11**(1):57–91.

West B, Jones NS. Endoscopy-negative, computed tomography-negative facial pain in a nasal clinic. *Laryngoscope* 2001;**111**:581–6.

Olesen J et al. The International Classification of Headache Disorders (2nd edn). *Cephalgia* 2004;**24** Suppl 1:1–160.

Woodford TM, Jones NS. In *Scott-Brown's Otorhinolaryngology, Head and Neck Surgery*, Vol. 3, Part 13, Chapter 135:1718–28 (ed. M. Gleeson), Arnold-Hodder, London, 2008.

CHAPTER 11

Paranasal Sinus Disease

Derek Skinner

Royal Shrewsbury Hospital, Shrewsbury, UK

OVERVIEW

- Chronic rhinosinusitis with or without polyposis is diagnosed by considering the history and examining the nose with a nasendoscope
- Coronal CT scanning is the imaging investigation of choice for rhinosinusitis particularly where surgical treatment is being considered
- Medical therapy for chronic rhinosinusitis with or without polyposis normally includes nasal douching with intra-nasal steroids for longer term maintenance therapy and the intermittent use of systemic steroids and macrolide antibiotics regimes
- Nasal polyposis is usually bilateral, unilateral polyposis may indicate a neoplasm rather than benign polyposis
- FESS surgery is the surgical approach of choice for treatment of refractory chronic rhinosinusitis

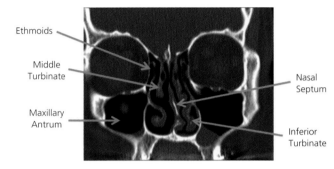

Figure 11.1 Nasal cavity with lateral wall clefts as seen on coronal CT scan.

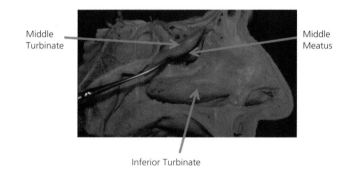

Figure 11.2 Lateral wall of nasal cavity.

Anatomy and physiology

The paranasal sinuses are air spaces within the bony facial skeleton with ventilation and drainage channels communicating with cleft-like spaces within the lateral wall of the nasal cavity (Figure 11.1). At birth, the ethmoidal sinuses are relatively well developed with 2–3 cells evident, the maxillary sinuses reach full size after the eruption of the secondary dentition, the frontal sinuses increase in development from 8 years old and the sphenoid sinuses develops from 3 years of age. All the paranasal sinuses continue to develop until the age of 18–20 years. About 5% of patients may not develop frontal sinuses as a normal variation.

The paranasal sinuses drain into cleft-like air spaces within the lateral wall of the nasal cavity. These lie beneath and lateral to the middle turbinate and the superior turbinate and are known as middle and superior meati. The normal mucus produced by the mucosal lining of the nose and paranasal sinuses is transported through the meati to the posterior aspect of the nose and nasopharynx; this is an active process controlled by the mucociliary system,

ABC of Ear, Nose and Throat, Sixth Edition.
Edited by Harold Ludman and Patrick J. Bradley.
© 2013 John Wiley & Sons, Ltd. Published 2013 by John Wiley & Sons, Ltd.

which is an integral part of the respiratory mucosa lining the nose and paranasal sinuses. The maxillary antra, frontal sinuses and anterior ethmoidal sinuses drain into the middle meatal region and the posterior ethmoid and sphenoid sinuses drain into the superior meatus and spheno-ethmoidal recess region (Figure 11.2). The naso-lacrimal duct drains the lacrimal sac into the inferior meatus anteriorly.

The exact function of the paranasal sinuses is unclear, however, these air spaces allow expansion of the facial skeleton to produce our recognisable facial features and may also act as a 'crumple zone' for facial trauma, so that the cranial cavity is adequately protected.

The osteomeatal complex (OMC) is an area comprising the middle turbinate medially and the mucosal-lined clefts and recesses of the maxillary antrum laterally. This is a critical area which must remain clear to allow adequate drainage of mucus from the maxillary antrum, anterior ethmoids and frontal sinuses. OMC obstruction, due to mucosal oedema, causes drainage obstruction from the sinuses, subsequently producing mucosal stasis and infection with acute and subsequent chronic rhinosinusitis.

The mucociliary mechanism within the paranasal sinuses and nasal cavity is of considerable importance to the health of the paranasal sinuses. It includes the pseudostratified ciliated mucosal lining – respiratory mucosa – with the overlying mucus, which is secreted by the seromucinous glands and mucosal goblet cells within the mucosa. The mucus forms two layers, a gel layer (viscous mucus blanket) which overlies a sol layer (thin mucus, bathing the cilia) and which allows movement of the viscous blanket of mucus through the sinuses into the lateral nasal wall clefts and subsequently into the nose and nasopharynx. The mucociliary system produces pathways within the paranasal sinuses and nasal cavities which are genetically predetermined and cannot be rerouted, thus allowing pathways of mucus to flow through the paranasal sinuses and nose. It is this mucociliary mechanism that fails in cystic fibrosis (due to excessive mucus viscosity), and in primary ciliary dyskinetic disorders (ciliary dysmotility), for example Young's syndrome. The mucus blanket may also become static due to acute infections, allergy, drugs and temporarily after nasal/sinus surgery. Subsequent stasis of the mucus blanket predisposes to acute and chronic rhinosinusitis.

Nose and paranasal sinus examination

Anterior rhinoscopy: This is (Figure 11.3) normally undertaken with a nasal speculum and allows a view of the anterior third of the nasal cavity. However, only a relatively limited view of the lateral nasal wall is possible. In children this can be achieved by pushing the nasal tip upwards to reveal the anterior nasal cavity.

Posterior rhinoscopy: This is achieved using a post-nasal mirror in conjunction with depression of the tongue. This provides a limited view of the nasopharynx and posterior aspect of the nasal cavity.

Nasendoscopy: This is performed with a narrow (2–4 mm diameter) rigid or flexible endoscope with or without surface anaesthesia/decongestion as a nasal spray and provides an excellent view of all the nasal cavity and the nasopharynx (Figure 11.4).

Sinoscopy: This is achieved by direct access to the specific sinus by puncture into the sinus cavity with a trocar and cannula and

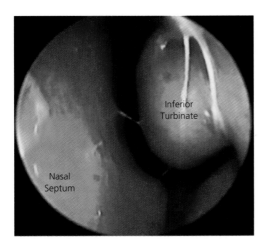

Figure 11.3 Anterior rhinoscopy, view in to left side nose.

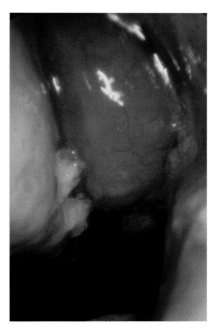

Figure 11.4 Nasal polyp in the middle meatus of a left side nose, as seen with a nasendoscope.

then subsequent insertion of a rigid endoscope, either with local or general anaesthesia and provides a full view of the specific sinus, usually the maxillary antrum.

Rhinosinusitis

Patients with rhinitic or sinusitic conditions normally would have similar mucosal changes within the nose and paranasal sinuses, hence the use of the term rhinosinusitis. There can be a dominance of symptoms arising from the nose or from the paranasal sinuses.

Symptoms and definitions of rhinosinusitis

Rhinosinusitis is considered an inflammation of the nose and paranasal sinus mucosa where two or more symptoms are evident. The main symptoms include nasal blockage or congestion and anterior or posterior nasal discharge; and facial pain or pressure, reduction or loss of sense of smell. Further symptoms which may be evident are sneezing, watery rhinorrhoea, nasal/palatal itch and eye irritation. Symptoms which resolve within 12 weeks can be regarded as acute and symptoms which are present for more than 12 weeks can be regarded as chronic.

Aetiology of rhinosinusitis

Allergy

Allergic rhinosinusitis is normally regarded as perennial, seasonal or occupational. A good clinical history of the nasal symptoms will often elicit the particular antigen. Perennial rhinitis is most normally caused by house dust mite allergy (dermatophagoides pteronyssinus). Allergy to dog dander and cat salivary protein found on cat hairs can frequently produce allergies within the home all the year around. Seasonal allergic rhinitis is most commonly due to pollens including grass, tree and flowers, particularly in the late winter, spring and summer season. In the autumn, seasonal allergy to airborne mould spores is frequently seen, for example *Aspergillus*. Occupational rhinitis may be due to airborne allergens including newsprint. Allergic rhinitis normally produces quite marked mucosal oedema within the nose causing subsequent reduced ventilation and drainage within the paranasal sinuses, subsequently producing mucosal stasis and predisposing to infection. The allergy is a type 1 hypersensitivity reaction mediated by IgE. Allergen-specific IgE facilitates degranulation of the mast cells and subsequent release of histamine and similar inflammatory mediators within the nasal mucosa, which produce the symptoms of nasal blockage, sneezing, rhinorrhoea, palatal irritation and eye irritation.

Infection

Rhinosinusitic infections can be viral, bacterial or fungal in nature.

Viral

Viral rhinosinusitis, known as the common cold, can last for up to 7 days with symptoms related to nasal obstruction, rhinorrhoea and facial pain/headache due to the nasal congestion. Rhinoviruses and coronaviruses are most commonly implicated and again nasal/sinus mucosal oedema causes failure of ventilation and drainage within the paranasal sinuses with mucosal stasis and subsequent secondary bacterial infection. Viral infections may also act by causing ciliary paralysis which again reduces mucus clearance within the nose.

Bacterial infection

Acute infection within the paranasal sinuses is usually aerobic in nature, particularly with *Streptococcus pneumoniae*, *Haemophilus*, *Moraxella* and pneumococcus. Less commonly, anaerobic bacteria can be found and this type of infection more frequently causes serious complications due to acute sinusitis, for example orbital or intracranial infection. Conditions predisposing to bacterial rhinosinusitis include viral rhinosinusitis, allergy, cigarette smoking, drugs impeding mucociliary transport and airborne fumes/irritants. Symptoms for acute rhinosinusitis are given in Box 11.1 and treatment is outlined in Figure 11.5.

Box 11.1 Symptoms of acute rhinosinusitis

Sudden onset of two or more symptoms, one of which should be either:

- Nasal obstruction/blockage – unilateral or bilateral
- Nasal discharge – anterior and/or posterior
    +/− Facial pain/pressure
    +/− Reduced/lost sense of smell

There should be complete resolution between episodes, each episode <12 weeks duration

---

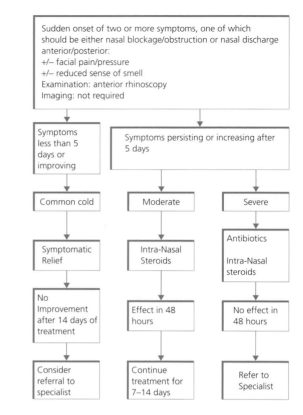

Immediate Referral to Specialist if:

Orbital Signs: Periorbital oedema, proptosis, diplopia, reduced vision Ophthalmoplegia

Intra-Cranial: Severe headache, meningism, frontal swelling

Figure 11.5 Treatment regime for acute rhinosinusitis in primary care.

Fungal sinusitis

Four main types of fungal sinusitis are noted. The most common forms include allergic fungal rhinosinusitis and fungal ball disease. These two forms of fungal sinusitis are non-invasive and with no immune system deficiency evident. Patients with allergic fungal rhinosinusitis normally have extensive bilateral intranasal polyposis and patients with fungal ball disease normally have symptoms related to a unilateral maxillary antrum, often with nasal obstruction and a bad smell within the nose. Chronic invasive sinus disease can have a slow indolent course causing erosion of the anterior skull base; however, angio-invasion can occur in the presence of the fulminant form of chronic invasive disease and this is particularly seen in immune-compromised patients. Only the chronic invasive disease requires antifungal agents. Fungal ball disease is normally treated with surgical removal of the fungal ball endoscopically and allergic fungal disease requires a combination of intranasal steroid sprays with nasal douching and occasional courses of systemic steroids.

Other forms of rhinosinusitis include non-allergic rhinitis with eosinophilia syndrome (NARES), vasomotor rhinitis, hormonal rhinitis, drug-induced rhinitis and granulomatous rhinosinusitis.

Almost 20% of patients with perennial nasal symptoms demonstrate eosinophilia within the nasal mucus without specific allergy evident, known as NARES.

Vasomotor rhinitis is due to an imbalance arising within the parasympathetic and sympathetic autonomic nervous system. A parasympathetic predominant condition would include profuse watery nasal secretion.

Hormonal rhinitis is often seen in pregnancy and at menarche as it is related to the menstrual cycle, particularly with oestrogenic activity causing nasal congestion. Drug-induced rhinitis is often seen due to beta-blockers, angiotensin-converting enzyme (ACE) inhibitors or with aspirin. The excessive use of beta-sympathomimetic amines as nasal decongestants can produce rebound congestion within the nose, otherwise known as rhinitis medicamentosa.

Specific conditions related to mucociliary dysfunction, including cystic fibrosis (mucoviscidosis), can produce thick mucus which is relatively static within the paranasal sinuses and nose and thus predisposes to infection and subsequent nasal polyposis, particularly in children. A similar effect can be produced by ciliary dyskinesia and this can be found in Young's syndrome and Kartagener's syndrome, again causing recurrent/persistent purulent mucus within the paranasal sinuses and nose. Granulomas and vasculitic conditions occurring within the nose and paranasal sinuses, for example sarcoidosis and Wegener's granulomatosis, often produce difficulties with marked crusting and infection within the nose and paranasal sinuses.

Chronic rhinosinusitis with nasal polyposis

Nasal polyposis is now regarded as a subtype of chronic rhinosinusitis and is found in up to 5% of the population, with some element of male predominance (Figure 11.4). The condition is frequently seen in adults over the age of 50 years, and up to 50% of patients have a strong family history. Nasal polyposis is seen in up to 20% of patients with asthma and in almost all patients with allergic fungal sinusitis. In patients with sensitivity to non-steroidal anti-inflammatory agents and who also have asthma, the incidence of nasal polyposis can rise to as much as 60%. This is sometimes known as Samter's triad. Nasal polyps are oedematous extensions of the intranasal and paranasal mucosa which contain large amounts of oedematous extracellular fluid. Nasal polyposis is most commonly bilateral in nature and any unilaterality of this condition would raise the suspicion of neoplasia. Patients with mucociliary dysfunction frequently produce nasal polyposis. Nasal polyposis in children with normal mucociliary function is exceedingly rare.

In young adults antrochoanal polyps may arise, which are large mucosal polyps arising from the maxillary antrum mucosa that extends into the nasal cavity and into the nasopharynx causing considerable nasal obstruction in this region (Figure 11.6).

Rhinosinusitis and nasal polyposis symptoms

Patients present with nasal obstruction which may be unilateral or bilateral with an associated sensation of congestion. There may be an anterior or postnasal drip which can be purulent or mucoid in nature and pain can arise within the face, often in the periorbital,

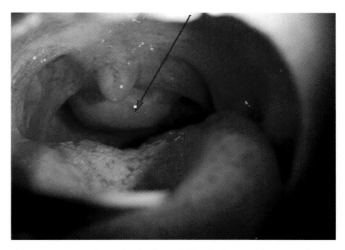

Figure 11.6 Antrochoanal polyp (arrow) lying in the nasopharynx and appearing in the oropharynx posterior to the soft palate.

bifrontal or infraorbital region (see Box 11.2). Purulent infection can often cause pain within the teeth of the upper jaw. Reduction or loss of sense of smell and taste is particularly associated with intranasal polyposis; however, sore throat, cough and dysphonia may be related to rhinosinusitis and malaise/fever may be present with more acute infection. Bleeding, facial pain and unilaterality of symptoms may sometimes suggest neoplasia and thus early surgical intervention with biopsy may be required. A full clinical history is essential to diagnose the antigenic aspects of allergic rhinosinusitis and this must include drug history, information on family pets and occupational exposure to airborne irritants.

Box 11.2 **Symptoms of chronic rhinosinusitis with or without nasal polyps**

Presence of two or more symptoms, one of which should be either;

- Nasal obstruction/blockage – unilateral or bilateral
- Nasal discharge – anterior and/or posterior

    +/– Facial pain/pressure
    +/– Reduced/lost sense of smell

Symptoms last for >12 weeks duration

Examination

Anterior rhinoscopy will reveal red congested inferior turbinates in the presence of an infective process, whereas the inferior turbinates are frequently pale or bluish and with a watery rhinorrhoea evident where allergy is suspected. Symptoms may be exacerbated by nasal septal deflections to one or other side and pus may be evident within the nose when bacterial infection is present. Nasal polyps are seen as pale grey translucent structures which have no tactile sensation within the polyps; however, palpation of the polyp may produce a sensation within the nose due to movement of the polyp on the more normal nasal mucosa. Nasendoscopy is essential to make the diagnosis.

Differential diagnosis

Anterior bifrontal headache and midface pain is frequently due to chronic tension face ache syndrome, atypical facial pain or migrainous syndromes. The clinical history around the nasal symptoms will make this more apparent.

Investigations

Allergy testing may be helpful for the diagnosis of seasonal or perennial rhinitis, particularly related to grass, tree and flower pollens, house dust mites, animal danders and bird feathers. This may be undertaken using a skin prick test or using radioallergosorbent test (RAST) blood tests for specific allergen IgE levels.

Blood tests

Eosinophilia is not seen due to allergic rhinitis alone, however blood testing to exclude Wegener's granulomatosis or sarcoidosis may be useful, particularly with anti-neutrophil cytoplasmic antibody (cANCA) and ACE.

Tests to measure mucociliary clearance within the nose and nasal mucosal biopsy may be useful when considering ciliary dyskinesia.

Imaging

Plain X-rays of the paranasal sinuses tend to be unhelpful with significant difficulties related to false positive and false negative findings. CT scanning of the paranasal sinuses in the coronal plane is now the standard imaging method for chronic rhinosinusitis, providing considerable anatomic detail for bone and soft tissues. MRI scanning may be a useful adjuvant scan where neoplasia or invasive fungal disease is being considered. MRI scanning undertaken for chronic rhinosinusitis will significantly overdiagnose this condition and will falsely demonstrate mucosal disease in the absence of clinical symptoms.

Complications of rhinosinusitis

Complications of rhinosinusitis occur in areas surrounding the paranasal sinuses, mainly the orbit and intracranial region. Preseptal orbital cellulitis can be seen as oedema within the eyelid region; however, this may progress to orbital cellulitis, which includes the orbital contents with suppuration causing an abscess within the orbit or in the periorbital tissues. Very rarely, cavernous sinus thrombus can occur. Orbital cellulitis and abscess cause increased intraorbital pressure, and results in ischaemia to the optic nerve and retina, which if not reversed can result in permanent damage to vision. Infection residing within the bones of the frontal region can occasionally be seen as an osteomyelitis and this may spread into the extradural or subdural space causing intracranial complications with the spread of infection through thrombosis within the venous system of the anterior skull region. Intracerebral abscess can subsequently occur due to further metastatic infective spread.

Treatment of chronic rhinosinusitis

Medical

Combinations of nasal douching, intranasal steroid sprays or drops, antihistamines, systemic steroids, antibiotics and especially

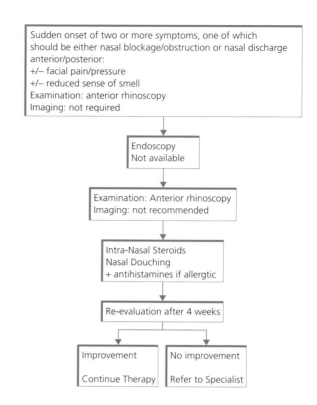

Immediate Referral to Specialist if:

Orbital Signs: Periorbital oedema, proptosis, diplopia, reduced vision Ophthalmoplegia

Intra-Cranial: Severe headache, meningism, frontal swelling

Figure 11.7 Treatment regime for chronic rhinosinusitis in primary care.

macrolide antibiotics may be required for treatment. Specific treatment algorithms are available with a good evidence base. These are illustrated in Figures 11.7, 11.8 and 11.9.

Surgery

Historically surgery has been undertaken using sinus lavage in various forms, sometimes known as antral washouts or lavage. This form treatment was effective for more acute-based infections but seldom curative for chronic disease.

Current practice would normally include the use of functional endoscopic sinus surgery (FESS) whereby the main disease area can be assessed and restoration of the ventilation and drainage systems of the paranasal sinuses achieved. Removal of polyps aids restoration of the mucociliary clearance, thus reversing the underlying cause for chronic rhinosinusitis. Endoscopic surgery allows only the minimal removal of normal tissue from within the paranasal sinuses and therefore facilitates more rapid healing. The combination of endoscopic approaches and external approaches to the paranasal sinuses may still be required for very severe disease, particularly in the frontal region. Minor complications from endoscopic surgery occur in less than 2%, for example formation of intranasal adhesions, epiphora due to nasolacrimal duct damage and bruising in the periorbital region. Major complications occur

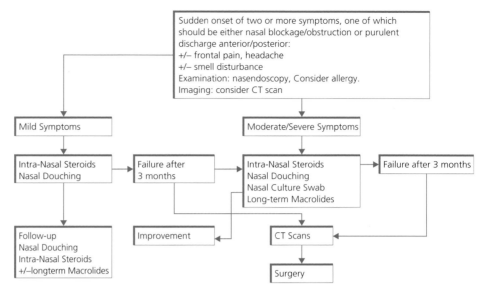

Figure 11.8 Treatment regime for chronic rhinosinusitis without polyposis in hospital.

Signs of complications may require surgical intervention.

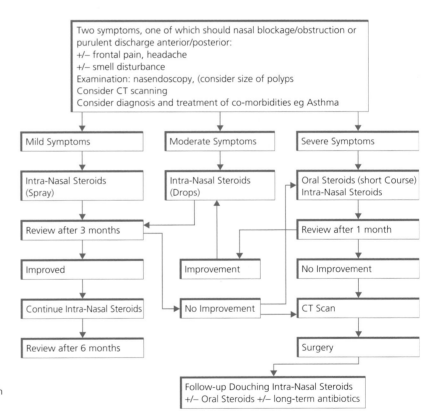

Figure 11.9 Treatment regime for chronic rhinosinusitis with polyposis in hospital.

in less than 0.5% and include diplopia, vision alteration, CSF leak, meningitis and intracranial injury.

Tumours of the paranasal sinuses

Malignant tumours of the paranasal sinuses are very rare. The commonest is squamous cell carcinoma and is commoner in patients exposed to nickel. Workers in furniture manufacture are also at risk of developing nasal adenocarcinoma if exposed to hardwoods for a protracted period of time.. There is a variable incidence reported in association with a benign tumour of the nasal cavity known as an inverted papilloma. Presentation may include unilateral nasal obstruction, facial pain, facial swelling and bloodstained nasal discharge. Management includes biopsy and imaging to aid staging. Treatment options include surgical excision and chemoradiotherapy.

Further reading

European position paper on rhinosinusitis and nasal polyposis. *Rhinology* 2007;Suppl 20:1–87.

Lund VJ (ed.). The nose and paranasal sinuses, in *Scott-Brown's Otorhinolaryngology, Head and Neck Surgery*, 7th edn, Vol. 2, Part 13. Hodder Arnold, 2008.

George AP, Skinner DW. Complications of sinus surgery – prevention and management. *J ENT Masterclass* (2010);**3**(1):26–31.

CHAPTER 12

Nasal Discharge

Andrew C. Swift

University Hospital Aintree, Liverpool, UK

OVERVIEW

- Nasal physiology, key sinonasal symptoms and conditions that cause nasal discharge in children and adults are considered
- Postnasal drip is just a symptom and not a disease – it may just reflect normal physiology
- A comprehensive history is of paramount importance in managing rhinological disease
- CT scans of sinuses should be requested only after adequate medical therapy of rhinosinusitis; plain sinus radiographs are no longer recommended
- The management of rhinosinusitis and urgent referral are both considered

Nasal discharge is one of a complex of sinonasal symptoms that we all have experienced at some stage. However, once it becomes predominant and persistent it can instigate a need for medical advice.

Normal physiology

It is important to understand the normal anatomy and physiology of the nose to enable a judgement to be made about the significance of the various clinical complaints that patients describe (Figure 12.1).

Mucus physiology

The nasal mucosa is a specialized dynamic lining that is covered with mucus (Figure 12.2). This mucus is part of the normal clearance mechanism that traps inhaled particles and is swept to the back of the nose where it flows down to the pharynx and is subsequently swallowed – a phenomenon known as mucociliary clearance. This normal physiology happens without awareness in most people. However, any alteration in awareness, mucus viscosity or volume may present with the classic symptom of so called 'post' nasal drip (*vida infra*).

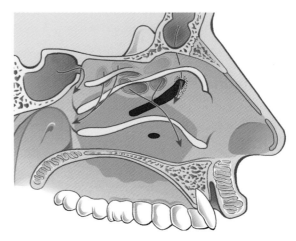

Figure 12.1 Anatomy of lateral nasal wall and sinus drainage pathways. (Used with permission from Thieme Publishers.)

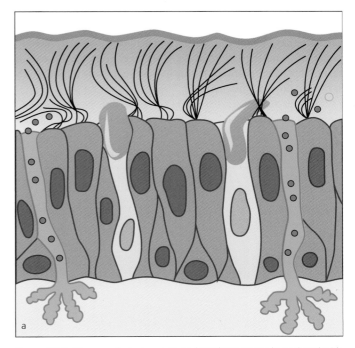

Figure 12.2 Diagram of nasal mucosa and overlying mucus layer. (Used with permission from Thieme Publishers.)

ABC of Ear, Nose and Throat, Sixth Edition.
Edited by Harold Ludman and Patrick J. Bradley.
© 2013 John Wiley & Sons, Ltd. Published 2013 by John Wiley & Sons, Ltd.

Mucosal physiology

The nasal mucosa itself is dynamic due to its specialised vascular structure, particularly over the inferior turbinates. The blood vessels control the degree of blood flow and thus vary the degree of congestion of the mucosa. This variation is determined centrally by the autonomic nervous system. In a healthy nose, this induces variation in the airflow between the two sides of the nose, over the course of several hours; a process known as the nasal cycle. It is therefore normal to have a better airflow on one side of the nose that changes to the other side with time. When this normal physiology is affected by rhinitis, patients complain of their nose being either blocked or runny, often in a cyclical sequence.

Congestion of the nasal mucosa is affected by nasal reflexes: the nose will feel more blocked whilst lying in a supine position, and lying on one side causes the downmost side of the nose to block. Rhinitis will exaggerate these reflex changes. Exercise will generally clear the nose.

Taking a sinonasal history

The first challenge when dealing with nasal discharge is to gain a clear understanding of the patient's actual symptoms. Since diagnosis normally relies on accurate history, it is best to use the words or terms that the patient recognises as part of what they actually experience.

In practice, a patient who is asked whether or not they have a nasal discharge often returns a blank or quizzical look. The use of descriptive terms and questions in a short conversation is therefore usually much more effective in eliciting the desired response. Patients should be asked whether their nose runs, drips or whether their nose is 'snotty' or if they need to sniff or blow their nose excessively. They should also be asked about mucus dripping into the throat, and whether they can cough or spit this out.

Once the history of discharge is established, the nature of the discharge can be explored. Key factors include the tenacity, colour, persistence and variation. Nasal discharge from the nostrils is termed anterior in contrast to mucus passing into the throat, which is termed posterior discharge.

Nasal discharge is a *normal* occurrence with head colds and usually this takes about 3 weeks to clear. The normal nose will also run temporarily in extreme cold conditions or when exposed to irritants.

Young children do not naturally blow their noses and their nasal airway is anatomically compromised. Nasal discharge is therefore a common and normal finding.

Excess mucus may be produced without any obvious underlying cause and patients may describe this as "catarrah". Discoloured or green-yellow mucus is consistent with chronic rhinosinusitis, but mucus that is not cleared quickly from the nose will become discoloured, particularly in the early morning after sleep.

The 'postnasal' drip

This term refers to the sensation of mucus at the back of the nose, but in most patients no abnormality can be seen.

There is a common misunderstanding that this mucus drips into the lower airway and then infects the lungs, but this is untrue. It is, however, true that inflammatory disorders of the nose are closely linked with those of the chest.

Chronic infection within the sinuses may cause a mucopurulent discharge into the nasopharynx. Mucus may be visible in the oropharynx but endoscopy of the nose is often required to see the more subtle findings of a mucus track.

Primary and associated sinonasal symptoms

Most patients with sinonasal disease complain of nasal obstruction and discharge is an important accompanying symptom. The other primary symptoms include facial discomfort/pain and loss of the sense of smell (Figure 12.3).

Discharge may be anterior from the nares or posterior when it induces throat clearing. In patients with rhinitis, discharge may alternate with obstruction.

The following symptoms need to be assessed in order to build up the sinonasal profile (Box 12.1).

The extended rhinological history

The nose can be affected by certain systemic conditions or be associated with disease of the lower respiratory tract. It is therefore important to recognize these problems and manage accordingly.

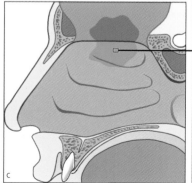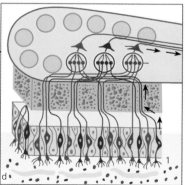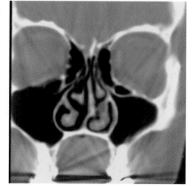

Figure 12.3 The olfactory mucosa and nerves. (Used with permission from Thieme Publishers.)

Clinical examination

Specialist examination of the nasal cavities has been transformed by endoscopy (Box 12.2). This is best done after applying a topical anaesthetic and decongestant. Rigid endoscopy provides a clear view that may demonstrate anatomical variants as well as subtle changes of sinus disease such as mucus tracks and polypoidal change (Figures 12.4 and 12.5, Box 12.3). Flexible endoscopy facilitates examination of the nasopharynx but can be extended to include the larynx and pharynx.

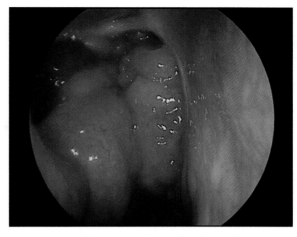

Figure 12.4 Severe polyposis in a patient with asthma and aspirin sensitivity.

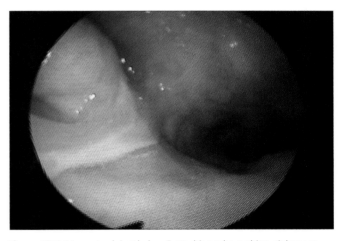

Figure 12.5 Mucus track just below Eustachian tube cushion, right nose.

Diagnostic red flags?

As with many conditions, the vast majority of patients who present with a nasal discharge have a common disorder that is not dangerous. However, occasionally some serious underlying pathology is hidden within this cohort of patients (Box 12.4). The two key conditions not to miss are:

1 Nasal tumour
2 Cerebrospinal fluid (CSF) rhinorrhoea.

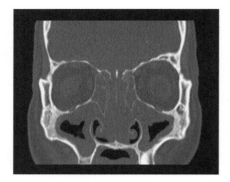

Figure 12.6 Multiplanar CT scan of patient in Figure 12.4.

Clinical investigation

Imaging

The most important means of imaging the sinuses is by a multiplanar CT scan (Figure 12.6). In patients with chronic rhinosinusitis, scans should only be requested after failure of symptoms to respond to adequate medical therapy.

Magnetic resonance scans may supplement the information from a CT sinus scan, but are normally only requested in special circumstances.

Allergy testing

Skin prick tests are used to identify atopy to various commonly inhaled allergens, including house dust mite, grass pollen, cat, dog and moulds.

Total IgE may be elevated in the atopic patient.

Serum specific IgE as assessed by radioallergoabsorbent tests (RAST) to specific inhaled allergens may be helpful, but tests are expensive.

Conditions that can cause nasal discharge in children

Adenoidal hypertrophy, rhinitis and rhinosinusitis

Most children presenting with nasal discharge have chronic rhinitis, rhinosinusitis or adenoidal hypertrophy. Rhinitis is easily recognised if the nasal mucosa is wet and congested. The appearance of the mucosa ranges from dusky red to pale pink: the latter is typical of the allergic nose. Allergy symptoms include sneezing, itching of the nose, eyes or roof of the mouth and throat, nasal rubbing and the so-called nasal salute.

Chronic rhinosinusitis without polyposis (CRSsNP) is more likely to be present if a mucopurulent discharge is present.

The clinical features of adenoidal hypertrophy include significant nasal obstruction, nasal discharge, loud snoring, nocturnal coughing, mouth breathing and adenoidal facies.

Uncommon causes of nasal discharge

In children

Primary ciliary dyskinesia – This is a rare autosomal recessive inherited condition that presents with nasal discharge from birth. Mucociliary clearance is impeded due immotile or dysfunctional cilia. Some children will have dextrocardia and bronchiectasis (Kartagener's syndrome).

Cystic fibrosis – Nasal polyps are uncommon in children, but when seen and when associated with long-term sinonasal symptoms, cystic fibrosis must be considered. The diagnosis is confirmed by a sweat test.

Rhinolith – A rhinolith that forms as a result of a long-term foreign body within the nasal cavity presents as a unilateral nasal discharge.

Choanal atresia – Bilateral choanal atresia, due to failure of the posterior choana to open, presents as an emergency shortly after birth. Unilateral atresia may only become apparent many years later as a persistent ipsilateral discharge. The diagnosis is confirmed by demonstrating complete lack of airflow through one side of the nose, failure to pass a soft rubber catheter through the nose, or endoscopy.

Tumours – Sinonasal tumours in children are rare but it is wise to maintain an index of suspicion.

Congenital swellings – Nasal encephaloceles, gliomas and dermoids are all rare but are more likely to present with obstruction and external swelling rather than discharge.

In adults

Rhinitis, rhinosinusitis and polyps – Rhinitis typically causes variable or alternating nasal obstruction and nasal discharge. The discharge may be watery, thick, tenacious or stringy. The latter is more likely to occur in rhinosinusitis, particularly if discoloured.

Acute rhinosinusitis normally follows head colds and is generally bilateral. The normal course of events is that the symptoms resolve after about 3 weeks (Box 12.5).

Nasal discharge can occur with chronic rhinosinusitis, either without nasal polyps (CRSsNP) or with (CRSwNP). A common error is to mistake congested inferior turbinates for nasal polyps, as they are easily visible in the anterior nares.

Watery rhinorrhoea in elderly patients, known as 'senile rhinitis', may occur due to autonomic factors as a result of age; the only effective treatment is an ipratropium nasal spray.

Less common causes of nasal discharge

Tumours

Inverted papilloma

Polypoidal growths within the nose are not always simple polyps, particularly if unilateral. The most common of these tumours is the inverted papilloma. This is a specific type of polypoid growth that normally arises in the ethmoid and presents with nasal obstruction with/without discharge. The appearance may look similar to an inflamed nasal polyp but they often have an irregular dull red surface (Figure 12.7). There is a small but definite association with malignancy and the diagnosis is confirmed by biopsy.

Malignant tumours

Malignant tumours within the nose are rare but vigilance is always required. Typical tumours include squamous cell carcinomas, adenocarcinomas, lymphomas and malignant melanomas (Figure 12.8). Unilateral symptoms of pain, obstruction and blood-stained discharge should alert suspicions.

Purulent maxillary sinusitis and fungal sinusitis

Infective maxillary sinusitis or a fungal infection may present with unilateral mucopurulent discharge. Fungal disease is characterised by greasy-looking mucoid crusts. Polypoidal tissue and discharge in the region of the middle meatus may be visible.

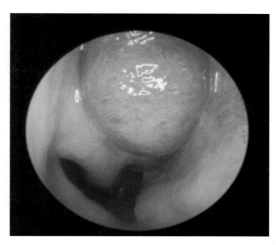

Figure 12.7 Inverted papilloma right nasal cavity.

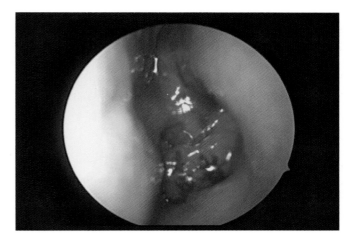

Figure 12.8 Malignant melanoma of left nasal cavity.

CSF rhinorrhoea

Unilateral watery discharge when leaning forwards, which stains the pillow with a halo is consistent with CSF rhinorrhoea. Patients will often describe the fluid as tasting salty. The presence of glucose by a glucose oxidase stick is consistent with CSF, although this has to be interpreted with caution. The most conclusive diagnostic test to confirm CSF in nasal fluid is beta-2 transferrin. Most CSF leaks are traumatic but some arise spontaneously. Both types carry a long-term risk of meningitis and should be identified and repaired. The defect is best localised by endoscopic exploration of the anterior skull base after injecting fluorescein intrathecally to stain the CSF orange.

Chronic granulomatous disease

Wegener's granulomatosis (WG) and sarcoidosis are systemic chronic inflammatory conditions that can affect the nose. Patients

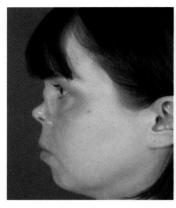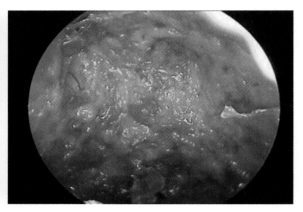

Figure 12.9 Saddle deformity and crusting in Wegener's granulomatosis.

with WG affecting the head and neck region often complain of unpleasant nasal discharge, and examination typically reveals extensive crusting. The disease is destructive and may cause massive perforation of the nasal septum and a saddle deformity (Figure 12.9). Failure to recognise and treat this condition can lead to death from renal failure.

Sarcoidosis is a multisystem disorder that causes marked nasal obstruction and mucorrhoea that is resistant to topical steroid medication. Skin rash, arthritis, pulmonary change and ophthalmic disorders should be sought.

How to manage nasal discharge

Investigation and management is determined by the diagnosis as based on the clinical features. The first line primary care management for commonly presenting sinonasal inflammatory conditions is shown in Box 12.2.

Conclusion

Rhinorrhoea may arise due to autonomic or pathological factors: topical nasal steroids are the main treatment for rhinosinusitis. Patients should be advised that they are safe for long-term use and instructed to use them daily over a period of 3 months for optimum effect.

Antibiotics should be reserved for acute purulent sinusitis or for chronic rhinosinusitis with mucopurulent discharge.

Any other disorder needs referral for specialist assessment and possible biopsy (Box 12.6).

Box 12.6 **When to refer for specialist assessment**

I. Urgent referral

- Blood-stained discharge (not epistaxis!)
- Unilateral polyp
- Unpleasant aroma from the nose
- Unilateral facial swelling and/or proptosis
- Unilateral watery rhinorrhoea in head down position

II. Routine referral

- Nasal obstruction that is unresponsive to topical nasal steroids
- Massive nasal polyposis
- Facial pain or discomfort
- Persistent mucopurulent discharge that recurs after medical treatment

Further reading

Behrbohm H, Kaschke O, Nawka T, Swift A (eds). *Ear Nose and Throat Diseases with Head and Neck Surgery*, 3rd edn, Chapter 2: Nose, nasal sinuses and face, pp. 116–227. Thieme, New York, 2009.

European position paper on rhinosinusitis and nasal polyposis. *Rhinology* 2007;Suppl 20:1–87.

Lund VJ (ed.). The nose and paranasal sinuses, in *Scott-Brown's Otorhinolaryngology, Head and Neck Surgery*, 7th edn, Vol. 2, Part 13. Hodder Arnold, 2008.

Roland NJ, McRae D, McCombe AW. *Key topics in Otorhinolaryngology*, 2nd edn, Bios Scientific Publishers, 2001.

Warner G, Burgess A, Patel S, Martinez-Devesa P, Corbridge R (eds). *Otolaryngology and Head and Neck Surgery, Oxford Specialist Handbooks in Surgery*. Oxford University Press, 2009.

CHAPTER 13

Epistaxis

Gerald W. McGarry

Glasgow Royal Infirmary, Glasgow, UK

OVERVIEW

- Epistaxis in children behaves differently from adult epistaxis
- Epistaxis in adults can be life threatening
- Unusually severe or persistent bleeding should initiate a search for secondary factors (e.g. haematological investigations)
- Primary and secondary epistaxis are different conditions requiring different management strategies
- Continued epistaxis following trauma must be referred to ENT
- Direct (bleeding point specific) therapy reduces hospital stay and morbidity
- Continued bleeding after insertion of a tampon should be seen as an indication to move to the next level of management, e.g.surgical ligation or embolisation

Epistaxis or nosebleeds occur in patients of any age and their severity can range from minor, nuisance bleeds to life-threatening bleeding requiring hospitalisation and surgical treatment. Epistaxis is the commonest reason for adult emergency admission to an ENT ward and it is a condition with a significant morbidity and risk of mortality. The quality of the initial and subsequent management of acute epistaxis can determine whether patients are effectively cured and discharged from hospital or whether they suffer continued bleeding and morbidity after invasive and ineffectual therapies (Figure 13.1).

The clinical types of epistaxis can be classified according to the scheme outlined in Box 13.1.

Box 13.1 **Clinical types of epistaxis**

- Primary (no obvious causal factor, the majority of cases)
- Secondary (due to an identifiable cause)
- Childhood
- Adult
- Acute
- Recurrent

ABC of Ear, Nose and Throat, Sixth Edition.
Edited by Harold Ludman and Patrick J. Bradley.
© 2013 John Wiley & Sons, Ltd. Published 2013 by John Wiley & Sons, Ltd.

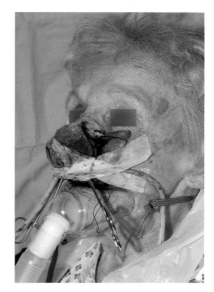

Figure 13.1 Patient showing the traumatic nature of poor management of an acute adult epistaxis. The nose has been packed with gauze, Foley catheters have been inserted and despite, or perhaps because of, this she continues to bleed but is now also hypoxic and severely traumatised. How not to do it!

Aetiology

The causes of epistaxis are poorly understood and most can be considered idiopathic. Cases can, however, be grouped broadly as either *primary* or *secondary*. The majority of bleeds fall into the primary category where no obvious cause is identified. Secondary epistaxis is due to a readily identifiable factor such as one of those outlined in Box 13.2. These secondary factors should always be checked for when taking the history. Rare causes such as tumours, hereditary haemorrhagic telangiectasia and juvenile nasopharyngeal angiofibroma are discussed later in this chapter but must be borne in mind as a high index of clinical suspicion is vital if these uncommon causes are not to be missed among the vast predominance of primary cases.

Childhood epistaxis

Nosebleeds are common in children of all ages and tend to be recurrent. Childhood epistaxis is mainly primary. They are often reported to occur at night and while the blood loss may seem alarming, it is seldom life threatening (a little blood goes a long way!). The commonest site of the bleeding vessel is on the anterior inferior part of the nasal septum in the highly vascular Little's area (this area contains Kiesselbach's vascular plexus). The exact aetiology is unclear but seems to involve mucosal inflammation and infection leading to blood vessel fragility. Nose picking may predispose to nasal vestibulitis, an infection caused by *Staphylococcus aureus*. Treatment of this chronic low-grade infection may explain the efficacy of chlorhexidine-neomycin creams in reducing the frequency of nosebleeds.

Management

If the child is seen while actively bleeding, first aid should be instituted by pinching the nostrils using the so called Hippocratic manoeuvre. Care should be taken to ensure that firm pressure is applied over Little's area by compressing the soft alar regions against the septum. Figure 13.2 demonstrates the correct and the surprisingly frequently observed incorrect application of this technique. Once the bleeding has stopped, the nose can be examined

gently and with a good source of illumination (a head light is ideal). If a bleeding point is seen, it can be sprayed with a local anaesthetic and vasoconstrictor agent (e.g. lignocaine and phenylephrine compound spray). Chemical cautery using silver nitrate on an applicator stick or diathermy with a bipolar electrode can then be applied to the vessel to control the bleed and to prevent recurrences. Care should be taken to apply the cautery only to the exact spot as a generalised application of silver nitrate can lead to further inflammation and infection and carries a risk of causing a septal perforation. Bilateral cautery should be avoided as it is seldom required and also increases the risk of a perforation. A course of chlorhexidine-neomycin cream is prescribed to prevent recurrence and promote epithelial healing. Nasal packs or tampons (see below) are almost never needed in children.

Adult primary epistaxis

This is the type of bleeding most frequently observed in hospital practice. Patients present with a sudden often severe nosebleed with no obvious causal factor. The bleeding is most commonly from the nasal septum but, unlike the bleeds encountered in children, is frequently from a more posteriorly placed artery. Bleeding from the lateral nasal wall is also occasionally observed and this can be very difficult to manage. The management is outlined in Figure 13.3 and ENT referral is mandatory in all but the most minor bleeds.

Initial first aid with the Hippocratic manoeuvre should be tried and a cannula inserted for venous access. In severe bleeds or where no specialist help is available, non-specialists will often resort to nasal packing. Nasal packing is a first line *indirect* treatment as it does not involve finding the bleeding point. In the past, ribbon gauze has been used to pack bleeding noses but this is a specialist technique which is seldom correctly applied. Incorrectly placed nasal packing is traumatic for the patient, damages the nasal mucosa, causes respiratory compromise and does nothing to stop the bleeding! Thus, non-specialists should try to avoid nasal

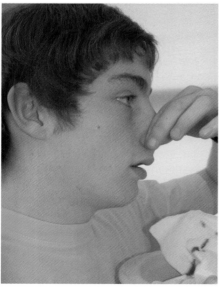

(a)

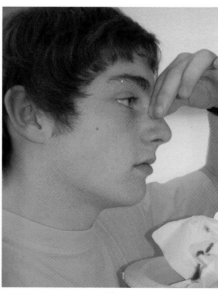

(b)

Figure 13.2 Correct (a) and incorrect (b) application of the Hippocratic manoeuvre. The soft part of the lower nose should be firmly compressed.

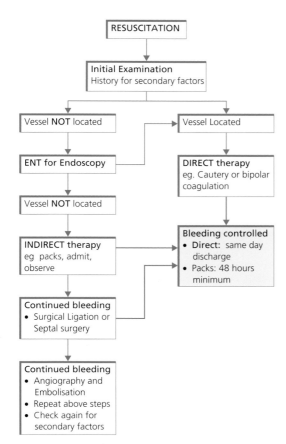

Figure 13.3 Management algorithm for all types of active epistaxis.

In some patients who are unsuitable for general anaesthesia or surgical intervention, vascular embolisation may be required. In this therapy an angiogram is used to identify the bleeding vessel and then its feeding branches are occluded by injection of thrombogenic material. Although effective, this procedure carries a slightly higher risk of complications than surgical intervention and it should be reserved for patients who are not fit for operation.

Secondary epistaxis

In this scenario the bleeding can be either recurrent minor or life-threateningly severe. The nosebleed is secondary to an identifiable cause, which may be pharmacological, haematological, traumatic, postsurgical or neoplastic (Box 13.2). It is vital to identify the underlying cause because the management of the bleeding requires correction of the causative factors in order to be effective, for example cautery will not work if the patient has taken too much Warfarin and the international normalised ratio (INR; usually 0.8–1.2) is 6.4!

Pharmacological

The commonest causes are use of prescribed or "over the counter" antiplatelet medications such as aspirin for cardiovascular prophylaxis or non-steroidal anti-inflammatory drugs (NSAID) used for pain control. The common combination of aspirin and clopidogrel in cardiac patients can present particular problems in management. Loss of control or overdose in patients on warfarin is another frequent clinical challenge. It is also important to ask about the use of so-called herbal medicines. Regular, even moderate, alcohol consumption has been shown to increase the risk of epistaxis in adults.

Haematological

Patients with thrombocytopenia due to alcoholic liver disease and those with blood dyscrasias due to haematological disorders can present with epistaxis which may be bilateral or from multiple sites. Occasionally the nosebleed is the initial problem that leads to the diagnosis of an underlying coagulopathy or blood dyscrasia. A careful history for other bleeding problems is required, but requesting a coagulation screen in all nosebleed patients is unhelpful.

Trauma

Epistaxis following craniofacial trauma is a serious condition requiring ENT assessment at an early stage. Nasal fractures can result in damage to the ethmoid bone with laceration of the anterior ethmoidal artery. Ethmoidal fractures commonly present with black eyes, nasal fracture dislocation with a broadened nasal dorsum and episodes of epistaxis which may be severe but intermittent after the injury. Such post-traumatic bleeds need early assessment and will often require surgery to ligate the bleeding vessel. Delayed rupture of the internal carotid artery is a rare but catastrophic consequence of skull base fracture which may be preceded by sentinel bleeds. Awareness of this rare complication can lead to early angiography with effective intervention in some cases.

packing. When all else fails, the correct use of a purpose-designed nasal tampon is much more likely to be beneficial than the excited ramming of gauze into a bleeding nose (Figure 13.1).

When faced with an acutely bleeding patient, ENT surgeons will seek to identify the bleeding vessel and treat it by *direct* means. Despite the initial alarm and continued bleeding, specialist examination using headlights, speculae and nasal endoscopes and suction apparatus will enable location of the majority of bleeding points. The commonest location for a bleeding vessel is on the nasal septum and so this area should be examined in detail first. If a bleeding vessel is identified, it should be controlled by direct application of cautery in the form of silver nitrate or, more effectively, by using specialist bipolar electrodiathermy devices if available. If a bleeding point remains hidden despite endoscopic examination, then packing may be required. Failure to achieve total control of the bleeding within the first 24 hours should be seen as an indication for referral to a specialist rhinologist for consideration of surgical intervention.

Surgical treatment may involve endoscopy under a general anaesthetic and diathermy of the bleeding point with or without septal surgery to improve access. If these measures fail, then the surgical procedure of choice for continued severe epistaxis is ligation of the blood supply. Endoscopic ligation of the main artery to the nasal cavity (the sphenopalatine artery) has been shown to achieve control of bleeding in over 95% of cases with few complications and allows patients to be discharged from hospital at an early stage. This operation should be available in most specialist ENT units.

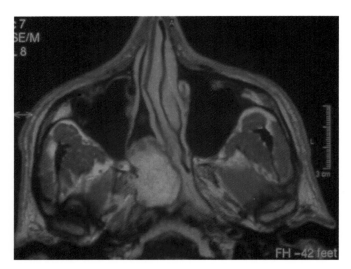

Figure 13.4 MRI scan showing juvenile nasopharyngeal angiofibroma in a 13-year-old boy who presented with epistaxis associated with unilateral nasal obstruction.

Bleeding following nasal operations is often due to surgical damage to vessels during the operation. Review by the operating surgeon will facilitate identification of the likely bleeding point. Following surgical reduction of the inferior turbinate, torrential epistaxis can be observed. This is due to bleeding from the inferior turbinate artery which is cut during the procedure. The management of this complication involves diathermy of the bleeding point, which may require further turbinate removal or, if this fails, sphenopalatine artery ligation (see below).

Neoplasia

Bleeding due to nasal tumours is uncommon and is usually associated with other symptoms. Unilateral bloodstained discharge with unilateral nasal obstruction should be seen as an indication for urgent ENT referral as nasal tumours can often present in this way. Unilateral nasal obstruction associated with epistaxis in a pubertal or adolescent male should raise the possibility of juvenile nasopharyngeal angiofibroma. This is a rare, highly vascular tumour which is diagnosed on nasal endoscopy and MRI scanning (Figure 13.4).

Management

In all cases the management follows the scheme set out in Figure 13.2. The essential point is that bleeding will be harder to control until the underlying cause has been addressed. Early consultation with haematologists and correction of any abnormality of haemostatic function (e.g. with platelet transfusions) may be required. Warfarin should not be reversed or withheld without first consulting with cardiologists and this is especially important in patients with prosthetic heart valves or stents. In patients with secondary epistaxis in whom *direct* bleeding-point specific therapies may not work, nasal packing can be used. As previously discussed, nasal packing should be seen as a temporary measure until specialist ENT help can be summoned. The most frequent form of packing used by non-specialists consists of an expandable foam tampon which is inserted gently along the floor of the nasal cavity. It is vital that the direction of tampon insertion is horizontal and parallel to the plane of the hard palate as attempts to stick things "up" into the nose will cause more trauma and bleeding and is potentially dangerous (Figure 13.5).

Hereditary haemorrhagic telangiectasia

This is a rare autosomal dominant inherited condition which shows variable penetrance and atavistic traits. It can present at any time in life but it commonly presents in early adult life with a history of severe recurrent epistaxis. Diagnosis is achieved when clinical suspicion leads to identification of the telltale telangiectases on the mucosal surfaces of the oral cavity and lips (Figure 13.6). Patients will often also have anaemia as a result of hidden blood loss

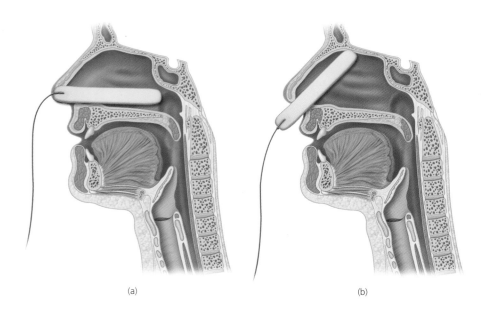

(a) (b)

Figure 13.5 Correct (a) and incorrect (b) directions for inserting a nasal tampon. In general tampons and packing should be inserted along a nasal cavity and not up a nose.

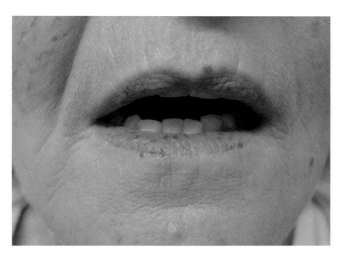

Figure 13.6 Patient with recurrent nosebleeds exhibiting the telltale signs of hereditary haemorrhagic telangiectasia.

from telangiectases in the gastrointestinal tract. The nose bleeds become more frequent with time and, while they may respond to cautery, they often require surgical intervention in the form of laser coagulation or skin grafts to the septum. In severe cases, surgical closure of the nasal cavity (Young's procedure) is an effective but drastic therapy.

Conclusion

Epistaxis is the most commonly encountered ENT emergency and, while it can often be difficult to control the bleeding, most cases will respond to logical stepwise management. The management steps are summarised in Boxes 13.3 and 13.4. Avoidance of nasal packing in favour of direct cautery to bleeding points allows more efficacious, cost-effective and safer outcomes to be achieved. The commonest cause of death in epistaxis patients is not catastrophic haemorrhage but more often repeated smaller bleeds which occur despite ineffectual treatment such as badly inserted packing. In this scenario, the continued lack of haemostatic control leads to anaemia, hypovolaemia and eventual cardiac ischaemia. This situation is best avoided by a proactive strategy aiming to locate and control the bleeding vessels. Any significant bleed, and certainly any case requiring a nasal pack or tampon, should be seen by the ENT emergency team. In patients who continue to bleed and do not have an easily identifiable bleeding point, an early decision

to proceed to operation is often a life saver. In addition to the therapeutic advantages of a proactive management strategy there are sound health economic reasons to ensure early control of bleeding as this shortens hospital stay, prevents re-bleeding and reduces treatment-related complications.

Box 13.3 Management guidelines for recurrent nosebleeds

- History (frequency, duration and enquire for secondary causes)
- Examine with headlight (look for vestibulitis or an obvious prominent bleeding point, remember to check for signs of HHT)
- Obvious vestibulitis should be treated with chlorhexidine-neomycin cream
- Obvious bleeding points or prominent vessels should be treated with cautery or bipolar diathermy followed by a course of chlorhexidine–neomycin cream
- Refer those with unilateral obstruction and blood stained discharge

---

Box 13.4 Management guidelines for the acutely bleeding patient

- **First aid**: Hippocratic manoeuvre, IV access, resuscitate
- **History**: enquire for and aim to address secondary factors
- **Examine with headlight and suction look for bleeding point**: can it be cauterised?
- **Continued bleeding?**: insert tampon and refer to ENT immediately

---

Further reading

Calder N, Kang S, Fraser L, *et al*. A double blind randomised controlled trial of management of recurrent nosebleeds in children. *Otolaryngol Head Neck Surg* 2009;**140**:670–4.

McGarry GW. Epistaxis, in *Scott-Brown's Otolaryngology*, 7th edn, Chapter 126 (ed. M. Gleeson). Oxford University Press, 2008.

McGarry GW. *Nosebleeds in Children. BMJ Clinical Evidence.* BMJ Publishing Group, 2011.

Melia L, McGarry GW. Epistaxis: update on management. *Curr Opin Otolaryngol Head Neck Surg* 2011;**19**:30–5.

Pearson BW. Epistaxis: some observations on conservative management. *J Laryngol Otol* 1983;**8**(Suppl):115–9.

CHAPTER 14

Nasal Obstruction and Smell Disorders

Desmond A. Nunez

University of British Columbia, Vancouver General Hospital, Vancouver, BC, Canada

OVERVIEW

- Nasal obstruction is a common presenting symptom for the entire range of pathological conditions of the nose. An approach to diagnosis starts with obtaining from the general medical history details of family, past or present history indicative of allergic disease, features of an upper respiratory tract infection and medications used, prescribed or illicit

- Anosmia or complete loss of smell is rare. Reduced or diminished sense of smell, hyposmia, is more common, and when due to a secondary conductive blockage usually responds well to surgery coupled with steroid medication

- The commonest nasal swelling is an enlargement of the proximal end of the inferior turbinate, that may be engorged by physiological and pathological disorders

- There is limited correlation between the severity of the septal deviation and the degree of nasal blockage

- The treatment of nasal polyposis can be medical, surgical or most usually a combination of both. Anti-inflammatory steroid therapy is a mainstay of treatment and best applied topically either in the form of a nasal spray or drops. Systemic steroids are prescribed in short courses to improve symptom control or as an adjunct to surgical treatment.

- Chronic rhinosinusitis is an inflammatory condition of the nose and paranasal sinuses with symptoms lasting for 12 weeks or more, affecting adult men and women equally, the diagnosis being made most commonly on symptoms

Symptoms

Nasal obstruction is a common presenting symptom for the entire range of pathological conditions of the nose. The key to arriving at a diagnosis is based as much on the associated symptoms as it is on the presentation and temporal characteristics of the nasal obstruction. An approach to diagnosis starts with obtaining from the general medical history details of family, past or present history indicative of allergic disease e.g. atopic dermatitis in childhood (allergy), features of an upper respiratory tract infection and medications used – prescribed or illicit. Many drugs can cause nasal obstruction, such as excessive use of topical vasoconstrictors in the nose.

The history should then focus on the presenting symptom of nasal obstruction and seek to determine:

- Onset of the nasal blockage – Is it sudden or gradual?
- The presence of precipitating or relieving factors – Is it triggered by exposure to perfume, suggestive of vasomotor rhinitis or following a nasal injury?
- Localisation – Is it bilateral or unilateral?
- Temporal characteristics – Is it persistent or intermittent?

Smell disorders

Anosmia – the complete loss of smell – is rare. The most common presentation of olfactory disturbance is hyposmia or a reduction in olfactory acuity. The olfactory sensory epithelium is located in the olfactory cleft in the upper reaches of the nasal cavity. The sensory cells are ciliated and contain odorant specific receptors. These cells synapse with the olfactory bulb in the forebrain by dendritic processes which traverse through the bony perforations of the cribriform plate (Figure 14.1). The binding of a specific odorant molecule with its receptor triggers depolarisation of the sensory cell and generation of an action potential that is transmitted along the olfactory pathways to the brain.

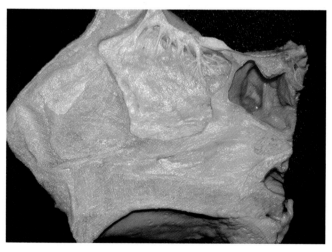

Figure 14.1 The olfactory fibres are shown in relation to the cribriform plate at the skull base.

ABC of Ear, Nose and Throat, Sixth Edition.
Edited by Harold Ludman and Patrick J. Bradley.
© 2013 John Wiley & Sons, Ltd. Published 2013 by John Wiley & Sons, Ltd.

A number of conditions can impair the olfactory process and these maybe categorised into:

Conductive block – This is due to nasal obstruction preventing the odorant molecule accessing the olfactory sensory cleft, for example excessive nasal mucosal oedema and secretions secondary to an upper respiratory tract infection or allergic rhinitis and nasal polyps.

Neurosensory – In these cases the olfactory receptors, neural pathway or olfactory cortex in the brain either singly or in combination are at fault, for example postviral, trauma-induced disruption of the pathway in a skull base fracture or higher centre dysfunction as in Parkinson's and Alzheimer's diseases.

Treatment and likely outcome

Investigation of the patient with a disorder of smell requires a complete nasal endoscopic evaluation in all cases. Potential causes of a conductive blockage of the olfactory system will either be diagnosed or excluded based on the endoscopic findings. An MRI scan of the brain is used to identify intracranial neurosensory causes of olfactory dysfunction such as intracranial extension of the rare olfactory neuroblastoma (a tumour that originates in the neuroepithelial cells of the cribriform plate). A CT scan is a better imaging investigation for tumours that arise in the nasal mucosa and then invade the olfactory sensory epithelium or for cases of head trauma. Cases of diminished smell acuity secondary to conductive block usually respond well to surgery coupled with steroids (e.g. nasal polyps). If the olfactory epithelium has been damaged – as in tumour invasion – or the connections between the olfactory bulb and the olfactory sensory epithelium have been damaged secondary to trauma, then the prognosis for recovery is generally poor. However, up to 20% of patients show spontaneous improvement with time after head injury or postviral olfactory loss, with higher reported rates the longer the follow-up.

Signs

The approach to examining a patient with nasal obstruction is identical to that used for assessing a patient with any other nasal symptom.

Commence with inspection of the nasal appearance, looking for signs of trauma, nasal deformity such as displacement of the nasal bones or an intranasal mass distending the nasal vestibule.

Proceed to anterior rhinoscopy or examination of the nasal passages with a bright light aided by the use of a nasal speculum to gently retract or open the alar cartilage. You should be supervised by an experienced clinician when first using a nasal speculum, as it is easy to over-distend the alar cartilage and cause the patient discomfort. The use of an otoscope with a wide gauge speculum is an alternative technique for the novice that is less likely to cause the patient discomfort. An otoscope is more likely to be available to students and clinicians practising outside a specialist environment. The otoscope will provide a light source and the otoscopic speculum retracts the alar cartilage.

Check the entrance of the nose for obvious obstructing masses. Look at the nasal septum. Is it distended in keeping with a septal

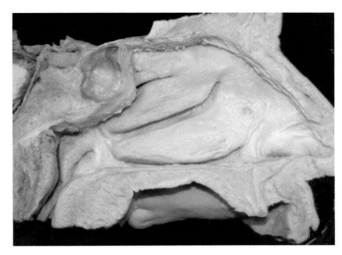

Figure 14.2 The lateral nasal wall showing the three turbinates.

haematoma or is it displaced into the nasal cavity on one side with a corresponding concavity on the opposite side, diagnostic of a septal deviation? The commonest nasal swelling to notice is the proximal end of the inferior turbinate (Figure 14.2). This bilateral structure can be alarmingly swollen and red leading to nasal obstruction in patients with a viral rhinitis associated with the common cold, or classically pale blue and boggy in allergic rhinitis.

When assessing nasal obstruction you should be aware that the most constricted part of the nasal airway is the region termed the nasal valve. This is a space bounded by the nasal septum medially, the medial surface of the anterior end of the inferior turbinate and distal end of the upper lateral cartilage laterally, and the floor of the nose inferiorly (Figure 14.3). The cross-sectional

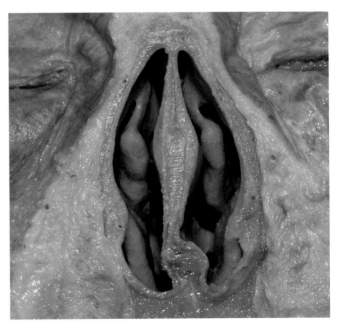

Figure 14.3 The nasal valve region in a cadaver. The walls of the valve namely the lower lateral nasal cartilages, nasal septum and nasal floor are demonstrated but not the medial surface of the inferior turbinate on this section.

area of the nasal valve is not static but varies inversely mostly with the size of the inferior turbinate and the degree of nasal septal mucosal congestion. The cross-sectional area is reduced not only by pathological conditions that lead to inflammation of the nasal turbinates but most commonly by the physiological nasal cycle.

The nasal cycle describes a 1- to 5-hour fluctuating alteration in the cross-sectional area of the nasal valve with both nares operating out of phase. Therefore, when the left nasal valve is constricted, the right is dilated and vice versa. The cycle is under the control of the autonomic nervous system but is abolished in the "flight and fright response" and blunted in inflammatory disease.

The patency of the nasal airway should be assessed as part of the clinical examination. Simple ways of doing so include observing the misting of a cold spatula placed at the entrance to the nasal passages as the patient is asked to quietly expire through the nose.

Diagnostic conditions

Nasal septal deviation

This is a condition named after the examination finding of a nasal septum which lies more to one side, deviated and resulting in obstruction or blockage of one or both nasal airways! It is a common cause of nasal obstruction in the Caucasian type nose but rare in racial groups with wider nasal bases (the distance between the left and right alar rims at the entrance to the nose). There is limited correlation between the severity of the septal deviation and the degree of nasal blockage. It affects both sexes equally and can present at any age. There is often no history of preceding trauma. The distinguishing symptoms are unilateral, persistent nasal obstruction in the absence of nasal hypersecretion, facial pain or olfactory dysfunction. On examination, the restriction of the nasal valve secondary to the deviated nasal septum should be seen and there will be corresponding evidence of nasal obstruction.

In clinical practice it is not usual to undertake further investigations to make the diagnosis. Clinical management depends on weighing up the relative risks and benefits of surgical treatment. Septoplasty is the operation undertaken to treat this condition. The operation is undertaken through the nose and does not involve any external nasal incisions. The main risks are haemorrhage though this is seldom of a significant degree, nasal shape change due to changes in the support of the cartilage nasal pyramid and septal perforation. The latter, due to poor healing of the septum following surgery, is fortunately rare in the hands of an experienced otolaryngologist.

Choanal atresia

This is an uncommon congenital absence of the nasal airway at the back of the nose due to disordered embryological development of the nasal passages. The most severe form of the condition leads to complete nasal obstruction that is persistent and bilateral presenting at birth. Newborns are obligate nasal breathers and the diagnosis is usually made in the delivery suite when a nasal suction tube fails to pass into the pharynx through either naris. There may be a history of respiratory distress particularly related to meals. The child may tolerate the nasal obstruction when at rest but is unable to feed effectively with complete nasal obstruction. Examination must exclude other anomalies of the oral cavity and pharynx such as a cleft palate.

The main investigation is a CT scan of the head to determine the nature and extent of the obstructive segment, as well as looking for other anomalies of the facial and skull bones. Usually the condition presents as an isolated non-syndromic anomaly. Treatment is endoscopic surgical choanoplasty with attention paid to preserving as much of the mucosal surfaces as possible to reduce the risk of re-stenosis. Indwelling nasal splints are sometimes used.

The prevalence of unilateral atresia is unknown as it presents later and with less concerning symptoms than the bilateral choanal atresia. Typically it is diagnosed in an adult with unilateral rhinorrhoea and nasal obstruction. Investigation and treatment is similar to the bilateral condition.

Nasal polyps

Nasal polyposis is an acquired condition of the nasal and paranasal sinus mucosa, presenting as inflammatory pedunculated swellings of the mucosa originating from the ethmoid sinus and surrounding lateral nasal wall. The aetiology is inflammatory, usually secondary to long-standing rhinitis. The diagnosis is most commonly made in adults in the fourth to sixth decades of life. Men are slightly more commonly affected than women. The history will often be positive for asthma and allergic rhinitis. On questioning, patients will admit to a gradually increasing bilateral nasal obstruction, long-standing anosmia and rhinorrhoea. Enquire about aspirin allergy to exclude the Samter's triad syndrome of nasal polyps, asthma and aspirin allergy. Anterior rhinoscopy should reveal the classical appearance of pale intranasal masses obstructing both airways. The masses are non-tender, soft and mobile if palpated with a nasal probe.

A CT scan (Figure 14.4) of the paranasal sinuses is the usual investigation to exclude features of malignancy such as bone erosion

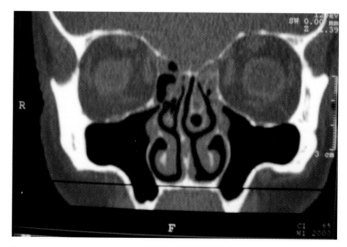

Figure 14.4 A Coronal CT scan of the paranasal sinuses illustrating marked ethmoid sinus inflammation and obstruction of the maxillary sinus outflow on the left. The middle turbinates are aereated and the left enlarged.

and the associated diagnosis of chronic rhinosinusitis. Allergy tests may be helpful if not already done. Treatment can be medical, surgical or most usually a combination of both. Anti-inflammatory steroid therapy is a mainstay of treatment. This is best applied topically either in the form of a nasal spray or drops. Systemic steroids are prescribed in short courses to improve symptom control or as an adjunct to surgical treatment. Surgery consists of endoscopic polypectomy alone or combined with endoscopic surgery of the paranasal sinuses.

Chronic rhinosinusitis

Chronic rhinosinusitis is an inflammatory condition of the nose and paranasal sinuses with symptoms lasting for 12 weeks or more. It is usually diagnosed in adult patients with men and women equally affected. The diagnosis relies mostly on the symptoms, solely so if using the American Academy of Otolaryngology Head and Neck Surgery Rhinosinusitis task force criteria. The symptoms are divided into major and minor and the diagnosis made if the patient has two major or one major and two minor symptoms. The European Academy of Allergology and Clinical Immunology requires the patient to have at least two symptoms (major or minor) and objective signs of sinus inflammation as demonstrated by middle meatal discharge (see Figure 14.5), nasal polyps or oedema on nasal endoscopy. The symptoms are shown in Table 14.1.

Treatment of chronic rhinosinusitis is initially medical and consists of:

- macrolide antibiotics for 12 weeks
- topical nasal steroid spray daily or twice daily
- regular nasal saline douches.

Patients who fail to improve with the above regime should be considered for functional endoscopic sinus surgery. There are several large case series that report the benefits of functional endoscopic sinus surgery with symptom improvement in 75% or

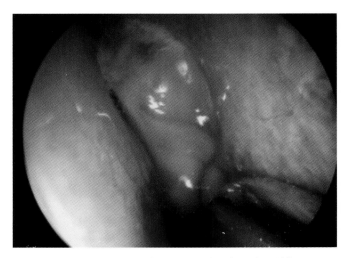

Figure 14.5 Endoscopic view of discharge arising from the middle meatus and surrounding the middle turbinate.

Table 14.1 The symptoms of chronic rhinosinusitis.

The major symptoms are	The minor symptoms are
Nasal obstruction	Halitosis
Facial congestion or pain	Headache
Anosmia or hyposmia	Ear ache (otalgia)
Nasal hypersecretion (rhinorrhoea and/or postnasal drip)	Tooth ache (dentalgia)
	Fatigue
	Cough

more of patients. There is as yet no randomised controlled trial evidence of the superiority of endoscopic sinus surgery to medical treatments, although surgery has been shown to be safe.

Investigations for nasal obstruction

There are no investigations commonly undertaken to assess the severity of nasal obstruction in the clinical setting. The investigations that exist are used for research purposes and are beyond the scope of an introductory text. If nasal obstruction is to be assessed in the clinical setting to demonstrate the efficacy of or need for treatment, patient symptom scores are preferred. An example of a validated questionnaire used in clinical practice is the Sinonasal Outcome Test (SNOT), a multi-item symptom question set.

The most useful investigation for differential diagnostic purposes is CT scanning of the nose and paranasal sinuses. A CT scan can help confirm a diagnosis of simple nasal polyps and differentiate it from intranasal malignancy.

Treatment

Nasal obstruction treatment depends on the cause. More than one condition can coexist and thus multiple treatments maybe required.

- The first-line medical treatment of nasal obstruction, in chronic inflammatory conditions consists of steroids that are delivered intranasally.
- Antihistamines are used in allergic rhinitis but have a greater effect on rhinorrhoea rather than nasal obstruction.
- Desensitisation is also an option in allergic disease and is once more being popularised because of the development of sublingually delivered oral medication that is more convenient for the patient and associated with a lower risk of anaphylaxis than the traditional course of desensitisation injections.
- Surgery is an effective treatment for nasal obstruction whether due to inflammatory or structural deformities. The most commonly undertaken surgical procedure for nasal obstruction includes septoplasty to treat a deviated nasal septum is highly effective with success rates of more than 80%. Inferior turbinectomy may be undertaken to treat rhinitis induced nasal obstruction resistant to medical treatments. This can take various forms, but all aim to reduce the size of the anterior ends of the inferior turbinates which contributes to the nasal valve. The various approaches differ in their success rates and complication profile.

Further reading

Khalil HS, Nunez DA. Functional endoscopic sinus surgery for chronic rhinosinusitis. *Cochrane Database Syst Rev* 2006;3:1–18.

Nunez DA, Bradley PJ. A randomised clinical trial of turbinectomy for compensatory turbinate hypertrophy in patients with anterior septal deviations. *Clin Otolaryngol* 2000;**25**:495–8.

Piccirillo JF, Merritt MG Jr, Richards ML. Psychometric and clinimetric validity of the 20-Item Sino-Nasal Outcome Test (SNOT-20). *Otolaryngol Head Neck Surg* 2002;**126**(1):41–7.

Thomas M, Yawn BP, Price D, Lund V, Mullol J, Fokkens W. European Position Paper on Rhinosinusitis and Nasal Polyps Group. EPOS Primary Care Guidelines: European Position Paper on the Primary Care Diagnosis and Management of Rhinosinusitis and Nasal Polyps 2007 - a summary. *Prim Care Respir J.* 2008;**17**:79–89.

Wilson DR, Torres LI, Durham SR. Sublingual immunotherapy for allergic rhinitis. *Cochrane Database Syst Rev.* 2003;2:CD002893.

CHAPTER 15

Facial Plastics

Patrick Walsh[1], Julian Rowe-Jones[2] and Simon Watts[3]

[1] Linacre Private Hospital, Hampton, VIC, Australia
[2] The Nose Clinic, The Guildford Clinic, Guildford, UK
[3] Brighton and Sussex University Hospital, Brighton, UK

OVERVIEW

- The benefits of facial plastic surgery are improved appearance and self-confidence, improved facial function and cure from neoplastic disease
- Septorhinoplasty is indicated for elective improvement of nasal function, aesthetic and nasal deformity
- Septoplasty alone may not restore nasal airway function and additional bony and external nasal cartilage surgery may be necessary
- The operating surgeon should be skilled in the management of both nasal form and nasal function
- There are three features that need to be surgically corrected with pinnaplasty: unfurling of the anti-helix, deep conchal bowl and/or prominent ear lobe(s)
- Non-melanotic skin tumours (NMSTs) are basal cell carcinoma (BCC) and cutaneous squamous cell carcinoma (cSCC)
- The treatment of BCC depends on size and histology
- The treatment of cSCC is surgical, and must be followed up to detect recurrence and possible cervical nodal metastases

---

Facial plastic surgery encompasses the management of patients requesting/requiring aesthetic change and/or correction of functional, traumatic and neoplastic disorders of the skin, soft tissues and facial skeleton. In both groups these conditions may be congenital or acquired.

In the neoplastic group of conditions, management of non-melanotic skin tumours (NMSTs) forms a sizeable part of our workload. Bearing this in mind, the NMSTs tend to be treated within the broad confines of multidisciplinary clinics. Treatment is surgical and non-surgical.

Facial plastic surgery is performed by ENT surgeons, maxillofacial surgeons, general and plastic surgeons, oculoplastic surgeons and dermatologists.

ABC of Ear, Nose and Throat, Sixth Edition.
Edited by Harold Ludman and Patrick J. Bradley.
© 2013 John Wiley & Sons, Ltd. Published 2013 by John Wiley & Sons, Ltd.

Septorhinoplasty

Nasal anatomy

The skeleton of the nose is formed in the upper third by of the paired nasal bones and ascending processes of maxilla. The mid third of the nose is formed by the upper lateral cartilages which attach to the nasal bones and to the cartilaginous septum and contribute to the internal valve. The lower lateral cartilages give support and shape to the nasal tip and external valve. Underlying and supporting these cartilages is the anterior cartilaginous part of the nasal septum, without which the caudal two-thirds of the nose would collapse (Figure 15.1). The type and thickness of the skin soft-tissue envelope contributes to nasal aesthetics and may influence the results of functional and aesthetic surgery.

Nasal function

The nasal valves

During inspiration the nasal valves are subject to collapsing forces due to the low pressure of the rapidly moving inspired air. The ability of the nares and external valve to withstand these collapsing forces depends upon the shape, resilience and position of the nasal tip cartilages. The internal valve normally measures approximately $10-15°$ and is measured between the septum medially and the caudal border of the upper lateral cartilage laterally. Surgery may require repositioning of these cartilages and grafting to strengthen and support them.

The septum and keystone area

The nasal septum is composed of the quadrilateral cartilage anteriorly, and the bony ethmoid plate, vomer and maxillary crest posteriorly and inferiorly. A deviation in the anterior and dorsal septal cartilage is a difficult surgical challenge as correction may require repositioning, reshaping and reconstruction of the entire cartilaginous septum and its associated upper lateral cartilages (Figure 15.2).

Assessment

The patency of the nasal airway and the aesthetic appearance of the nose should be considered in all patients even though the presenting complaint may relate more to one of these than the other. This is because an operation to correct an aesthetic anomaly may affect the

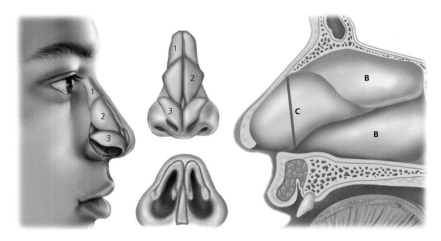

Figure 15.1 Left: Anatomy of the external nasal skeleton: 1, nasal bones; 2, upper lateral cartilages; 3, lower lateral cartilages; 4, septum (inside the nose). Right: Anatomy of the nasal septum: B, bone; C, cartilage, with the line of nasal support between keystone area superiorly and anterior nasal spine inferiorly shown in blue. (Copyrighted to The Nose Clinic.)

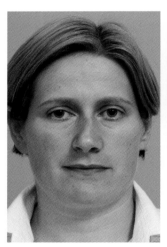
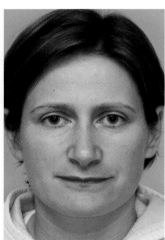
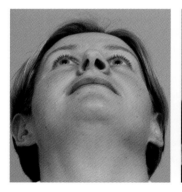
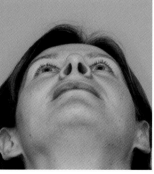

Figure 15.2 Preoperative (left) and postoperative (right) views of a patient with a twisted nose presenting with nasal obstruction due to combined deformity of the nasal bones, upper lateral cartilages and anterior septum. Relief of obstruction in this case requires septorhinoplasty. (Copyrighted to J Rowe-Jones.)

Table 15.1 Septorhinoplasty: indications and contraindications.

Indications	Contraindications
Acute saddle nose following trauma	Pre-primary school age
Functional: combined nasal and septal deformity causing obstruction	Severe co-morbid conditions
	Major psychiatric illness or personality disorder
Aesthetic	

Box 15.1 **Important features to note at consultation**

Nasal skeleton

- Assess the upper (bony) third, middle (cartilaginous) third and lower third (tip) of the nose for deformity
- Examine the nose from frontal, lateral, oblique and basal views (Figure 15.3)

Nasal valves

- Dimensions of internal and external valves
- Narrowing of the valve areas with inspiration

Nasal septum

- Malposition of the dorsal and caudal leading edges
- Twists, curves or other abnormalities of shape

Psychological

- Determine the primary concern of the patient and their expectations
- Exclude major psychological illness, body dysmorphia, and significant personality disorder

Postoperative care and complications

- An external splint is required for 1 week postoperation.
- The appearance of a haematoma of the septum or external nose requires surgical review. An untreated haematoma may lead to collapse of the nose.
- Cutaneous infections may lead to visible scarring and contracture and need aggressive treatment and review.
- Secondary haemorrhage can occur up to 2 weeks after surgery

architecture of the nasal valves, and an operation to alleviate nasal obstruction may necessitate alteration to the nasal bones, upper and/or lower lateral cartilages, and hence the appearance of the nose (Table 15.1).

Important features to note at consultation are given in Box 15.1.

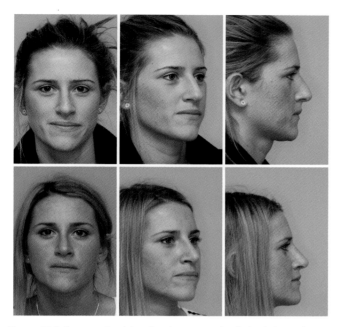

Figure 15.3 Pre-operative (above) and postoperative (below) views of a patient seeking cosmetic septorhinoplasty to correct her dorsal hump and her nasal tip. She has an asymmetric face with a nasal twist. Open approach enabled dorsal reduction, tip refinement and straightening of the nose. (Copyrighted to J Rowe-Jones.)

- Healing is protracted and patients often require support during this time. The final outcome of surgery may not be evident for 12 months or more.

Pinnaplasty

Prominent or "bat ears" can result in merciless teasing, which affects approximately 15% of the population and correction of this problem is very commonplace! The ideal age at which to undertake a pinnaplasty is preschool as the cartilage is still soft, allowing for easy remodelling.

Correction of a prominent pinna deformity by using the surgical techniques of pinnaplasty or otoplasty, has resulted in many different described and named approaches, suggesting that there is no single ideal technique to resolve all of the possible anatomical deformities. It is important to identify the defect(s) accurately before embarking on re-establishing the complex normal anatomy.

If the ears are obviously prominent at birth, they can be medialised with a head band for 3–4 weeks or a soft "pipe cleaner" type splint can be applied to help reform the anti-helix.

As with any potential aesthetic procedure, pre-operative photography is essential as it is a medicolegal requirement, plus it helps the surgeon to plan the procedure.

The procedure

This is usually performed under a general anaesthetic in children but local anaesthetic is a possibility in adult patients. There are three main potential deformities to address, namely unfurling of the anti-helix, deep conchal bowl and/or prominent ear lobe(s), each requiring different techniques to produce a reliable, lasting result (Figure 15.4).

Complications

Early complications are those of haematoma formation and infection, both of which result in excessive pain in the postoperative period. Both problems require immediate antibiotic therapy and the release of any trapped blood/serous fluid is essential to prevent a lasting deformity from developing.

Late complications include asymmetry and/or unfurling of the pinna, irregularity of cartilage edges, prolonged numbness and extrusion of deep sutures.

Non-melanoma skin tumours

There are two main groupings of NMST, namely basal cell carcinoma (BCC) and cutaneous squamous cell carcinoma (cSCC) (Table 15.2). The BCCs are further subdivided into superficial spreading and nodular subtypes which make up over 80% of all BCCs, but there is a more aggressive, morphoeic subgroup found

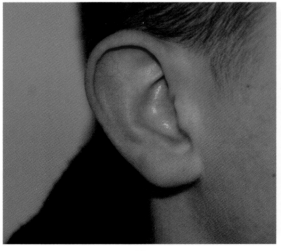

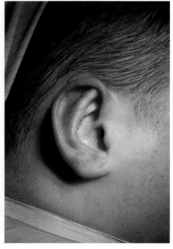

Figure 15.4 (a) Pre-operative pinnaplasty and (b) post-operative pinnaplasty.

(a)

(b)

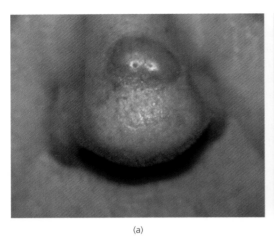
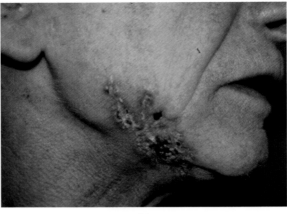

(a)   (b)

Figure 15.5 Typical examples of NMSTs: (a) basal cell carcinoma of the nose; (b) cutaneous squamous cell carcinoma.

Table 15.2 High risk features of local recurrence.

Basal cell carcinoma (BCC)	Cutaneous squamous cell carcinoma (cSCC)
Size >2cm	Size >2 cm
	Depth >4 mm thickness, Clark level V or beyond
Tumour site: the central face, around eyes nose lips and ears Poor definition of clinical margins	Site of primary: ear or non-hair-bearing lip, scalp
Histological subtype: micronodular, morphoeic, infiltrative, basosquamous Histological features of aggression: perineural and/or perivascular involvement	Histological features: perineural, lymphatic or vascular invasion: poorly differentiated or undifferentiated tumours
Failure of previous treatment Immunosuppression	Failure of previous treatment Immunosuppression

exclusively in the head and neck, the commonest single site being the nose. A morphoeic BCC behaves like a cSCC and thus requires treatment as if it were an SCC. Other locally destructive types of skin tumours include the micronodular, infiltrative and basosquamous (Figure 15.5).

The current policy for treatment of NMST within the GP community in the UK is very much dependent upon the individual GP concerned as some have basic dermatological skills. To this end, small (<5 mm) BCCs can, as a rule, be treated within the GP's surgery; referral to hospital specialists is encouraged for bigger lesions (Box 15.2). Most specialist institutions with a tertiary referral base will now run a multidisciplinary clinic with input from most practitioners treating NMSTs. This helps both specialists and GPs to discuss the management of complex or recurrent disease within a multidisciplinary setting.

Medical treatment

If an NMST is small (<5 mm) and does not involve the lip, eyelid or nose, then it can be destroyed using cautery or cryotherapy, resulting in crusting that heals with a pale and concaved area over 3 weeks. This approach is simple and can be performed as an office procedure, but the drawbacks are there is no histological confirmation of the diagnosis.

> **Box 15.2 Referral guidelines for suspected skin cancer**
>
> **Urgent referral**
>
> - Lesion suspected to be melanoma (excision in primary care should be avoided)
> - Non-healing keratinising or crusted tumours larger than 1 cm with significant induration on palpation; they are commonly found on the face, scalp or back of the hand with a documented expansion over 8 weeks
> - Patients who have had an organ transplant and develop new or growing cutaneous lesions as squamous cell carcinoma is common with immunosuppression but may be atypical and aggressive
> - Histological diagnosis of a squamous cell carcinoma
>
> **Non-urgent referral**
>
> - Basal cell carcinomas are slow growing, usually without significant expansion over 2 months, and usually occur on the face; if basal cell carcinoma is suspected, refer non-urgently
>
> **Investigations**
>
> - All pigmented lesions that are not viewed as suspicious of melanoma but are excised should have a lateral excision margin of 2 mm of clinically normal skin and cut to include subcutaneous fat in depth
> - Send all excised skin specimens for pathological examination
> - When referring a patient in whom an excised lesion has been diagnosed as malignant, send a copy of the pathology report with the referral correspondence

Radiotherapy can also be used with great success but it tends to be used for patients with large lesions who are unfit for surgery.

Photodynamic therapy may be used for patients with Bowens's disease (multiple low-risk superficial BCCs).

Topical 5% imiquimod, an immune response modifier, is effective in the treatment of small primary superficial BCCs (requires a license).

Surgical treatment

Most superficial spreading/nodular BCCs should be removed with a 2- to 3-mm margin to ensure >95% tumour-free margins. As excised tumours with a positive histological margin are extremely slow growing and there is a low risk of neck metastasis, controversy exists about their treatment, i.e. re-excision versus a "watch and wait" policy.

Morphoeic and large BCCs and cSCCs are excised with 4- to 5-mm margins. Follow-up for 5 years is important as 5% have the potential to metastasise to the neck. However, residual morphemic/SCC disease should be re-excised, as this tends to grow quickly and may spread to the neck.

Mohs' micrographic surgery (MMS) is a precise technique which combines staged resection with comprehensive histological examination of the surgical margin. Recommended in recurrent NMSC and those with adverse histological features, especially in anatomically critical sites. The main problems with this technique include the length of the procedure, the need for special equipment and training and the relatively high cost.

Management of regional metastases: the overall risk is 5% in NMST, but higher in aggressive high-risk tumours, those with adverse histological features such as poor differentiation or perineural infiltration, and tumours thicker than 4 mm. Referral to a head and neck clinic where surgery (neck dissection) is the primary mode of treatment for established nodal involvement and adjuvant radiotherapy improves survival in some risk cases.

Surgical principles

When faced with a facial defect after tumour removal, it is important to consider a few basic objectives:

- Which subunit of the face is the defect sited in and does that defect cross subunit boundaries? If there is a "cross-boundary defect" the boundary needs to be highlighted and respected when performing the reconstruction to preserve the cosmetic definition of that subunit.
- What is the three dimensional extent of the defect, is the tissue healthy (postradiotherapy, etc.) and is there exposed bone/cartilage? These considerations will not only help to define the *type* of reconstruction (e.g. a vascularised flap for exposed cartilage) but also the *extent* as more than one reconstructive modality is needed to close some defects (e.g. through-and-through nasal defects)
- Is the reconstruction going to impact on other dynamic structures (e.g. lips, eyelids, nostrils), as the vector of closure may be altered to avoid this?
- Have more than one surgical solution to closing a facial defect as occasionally things do not go as planned and a back-up plan is important. Don't become a "one-trick pony!"
- Lastly, regardless of the defect or your preconceptions, run through the *entire* reconstructive ladder (considering the most simple repair to the most complex) when considering your options and then include or exclude on the basis of sound surgical principles (Figure 15.6).

Primary closure

Ideally closure without tension is best as it will ensure a small, undistorted scar, but it is also desirable to place that scar within the

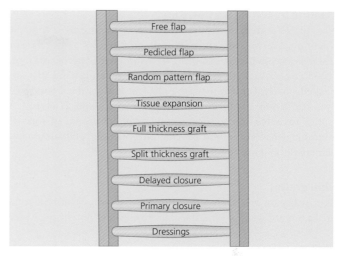

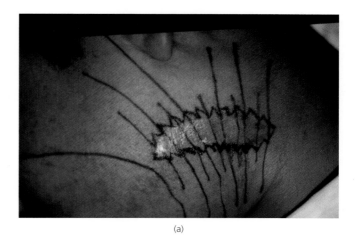

Figure 15.6 The reconstructive surgical ladder.

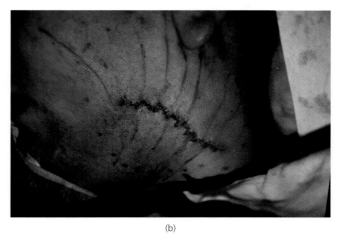

(a)

(b)

Figure 15.7 Cutaneous squamous cell carcinoma of the cheek/jaw: (a) pre-operative; (b) postoperative.

relaxed skin tension lines (RSTLs; Langer's lines) as this will help to disguise the scar within the naturally occurring folds of the face (wrinkles!). If this is not possible, creation of an irregular wound will tend to draw the eye less than a straight scar (Figure 15.7).

Healing by secondary intention

Not all facial defects require closure and healing by secondary intention is very useful. There are some golden rules: (a) the base of the defect needs to be clean with no exposed bone and/or cartilage, (b) The base also needs to contain viable, granulating tissue that can heal effectively, (c) it is inevitable that the base of the wound will "pucker" a little and fill out the defect somewhat and, as a result, it is thus advisable only to allow secondary intent healing in areas of concavity (medial canthus; conchal bowl; temple; philtrum; nasal alar crease) (Figure 15.8).

Skin grafts

Skin grafts are invariably a double-edged sword as skin reservoirs are in bountiful supply and thus easy to consider but, by their very nature, they have no guaranteed blood supply and their use thus needs to be carefully considered to accommodate this problem.

There are three types of skin graft to consider each having fairly specific indications.

Split thickness skin grafts (SSG)

The main advantage to SSG's is that there are numerous locations from which they can be harvested, the disadvantage is that they do not produce an aesthetically pleasing result long term and generally their use is thus limited on the face to very superficial grafting of the pale nasal side-wall or to gaining coverage of a large defect where there may be residual tumour that will show up quickly if it recurs (Figure 15.9).

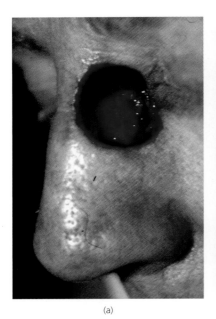
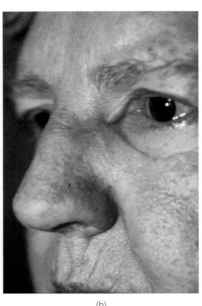

(a)   (b)

Figure 15.8 Lateral nose: (a) surgical defect; (b) post-healing by secondary intention.

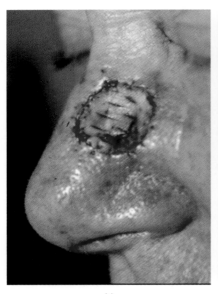
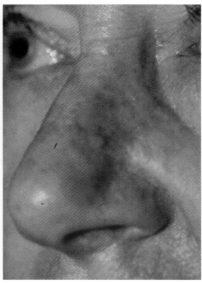

(a)   (b)

Figure 15.9 Healing by split skin grafting: (a) skin applied to defect; (b) post-healing effect.

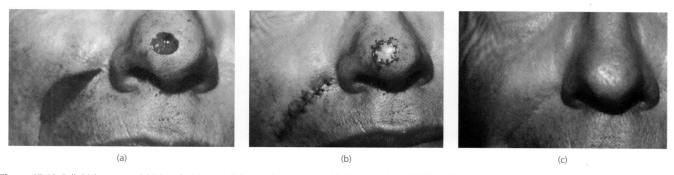

Figure 15.10 Full thickness nasolabial graft: (a) nasal defect and donor area; (b) closure of (nasolabial) defect and fixation of graft; (c) final cosmetic result.

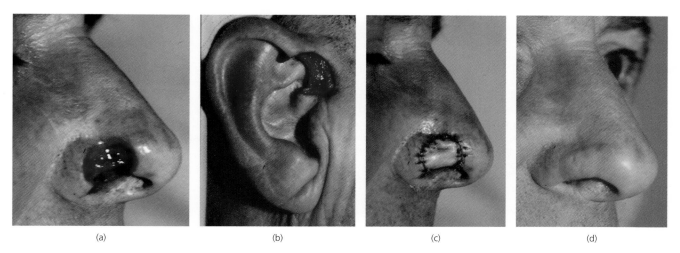

Figure 15.11 Use of composite graft technique: (a) alar defect; (b) donor graft defect; (c) graft sutured into alar defect; (d) final cosmetic result.

Full thickness

The reservoirs for these grafts are also multiple, the common sites for harvesting are the pre-auricular and postauricular areas, the supraclavicular area and the nasolabial crease. The skin from the nasolabial crease is particularly sebaceous and thick, which is useful for small nasal tip lesions (Figure 15.10).

Composite

Involvement of areas of the face such as the nasal ala or columella, composite skin grafts (skin grafts with cartilage or bone included) should be considered an option. The size of the defect for reconstruction should be no larger than 10 mm as the blood supply will simply not sustain the needs of the bulky graft tissue.

The most appropriate donor site for these grafts is the root of the helix as it provides robust support, plus it leaves behind a very small donor site defect (Figure 15.11).

Skin flaps

The advantage that skin flaps have over skin grafts is that they are vascularised, ensuring a better chance of viability. The vascular supply can be random in nature, with the flap relying on multiple, deep perforators, or it is derived from a named axial blood vessel, resulting in a much more robust, reliable surgical outcome.

When deciding what type of flap to use in the reconstruction, it is useful to classify them into either flaps that rotate around a pivotal point (rotational) or flaps that move along a linear axis (advancement). Whatever method of flap construction is decided upon, the key to a successful flap reconstruction is to identify where the areas of abundant skin are in close proximity to the defect and to use those to maximum benefit without distorting surrounding structures (Figure 15.12).

Microvascular free flaps (MVFF)

When large head and neck resections are undertaken, there is occasionally a loss of external skin or mucosa due to tumour involvement that is too significant in size to cover with a local flap. Such defects are ideally closed with a MVFF that has a guaranteed blood supply to ensure viability. The best known of the MVFFs is the radial free forearm flap based on the radial artery and antecubital veins. It is robust and provides a sizeable area of skin for coverage, but the donor area is unsightly as it is usually covered with a split skin graft. If bone is needed for a partial or full mandibular replacement, then some radius bone can be incorporated for this purpose.

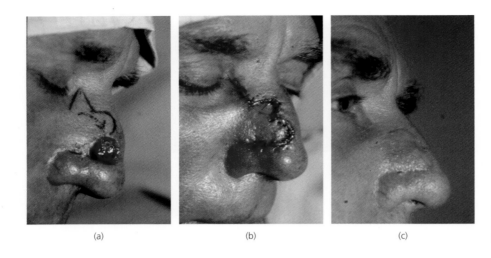

(a) (b) (c)

Figure 15.12 Use of a skin flap: (a) nasal BCC lesion with outline of rhomboid flap; (b) flap rotated into defect; (c) final cosmetic result.

Further reading

Bath-Hextall FJ, Perkins W, Bong J, Williams HC. Interventions for basal cell carcinoma of the skin. *Cochran Database Syst Rev* 2007;Issue 1:CD003412.

Motley R, Kersey P, Lawrence C, British Association of Dermatologists, British Association of Plastic Surgeons. Multiprofessional guidelines for the management of the patient with primary cutaneous squamous cell carcinoma. *Br J Plast Surg* 2003;**56**:85–91.

National Institute for Health and Clinical Excellence (2006) http://guidance.nice.org.uk/CSGSTIM (accessed 16 December 2011).

Telfer NR, Colver GB, Morton CA. Guidelines for the management of basal cell carcinoma. *Br J Dermatol* 2008;**159**:35–48.

Vauterin TJ, Veness MJ, Morgan GJ, Poulson MG, O'Brien CJ. Patterns of lymph node spread of cutaneous squamous cell carcinoma of the head and neck. *Head Neck* 2006;**28**:785–91.

CHAPTER 16

Throat Pain

William McKerrow[1] and Patrick J. Bradley[2]

[1]NHS Education for Scotland, Centre For Health Science, Inverness, UK
[2]Nottingham University Hospitals, Queen's Medical Centre Campus, Nottingham, UK

OVERVIEW

- Throat pain is a symptom most commonly seen in general practice or by hospital emergency departments usually in children and young adults although it can occur at any age

- When the symptom is chronic or recurrent, then the differential diagnosis may range from being a minor non-serious condition or be a sign of significant disease, such as a specific infective process or a throat cancer

- Worrying symptoms associated with throat pain, such as difficulty breathing, swallowing problems, the need to "clear the throat", bringing up blood and the presence of a swelling or a neck lump, should be investigated with urgency

- Infective processes if left untreated may develop into a local collection of pus or an abscess, most commonly the peritonsillar abscess or quinsy, but other more serious diagnoses include the parapharyngeal abscess and retropharyngeal abscess, which may be life-threatening if not recognised and treated effectively

Throat pain is a symptom most commonly seen in general practice or by hospital emergency departments, usually in children and young adults, although it can occur at any age. The symptom usually presents acutely, and is most often associated with an infective process – either viral or bacterial. When what seems to be a minor throat symptom with or without pain becomes chronic or recurrent, the range of diagnosis may be a "trivial" non-serious cause to becoming a "life and death" disease such as cancer or a specific infective process. A possible problem in diagnosis is the anatomical area to which the patient or parent is referring when they present with a painful throat. For the trained clinician with either a medical or a nursing background, the throat refers to the area called the pharynx, usually the oropharynx and the hypopharynx, and the term "pharyngitis" or "tonsillitis" is the assumed diagnosis. For patients, this term may be too restrictive. They may include areas such as the "mouth" and the "larynx" or "voice-box", or even any location within the neck and above the "collar-bone".

Persisting symptoms associated with throat pain, should alert the clinician to consider a "more serious" diagnosis, more so if

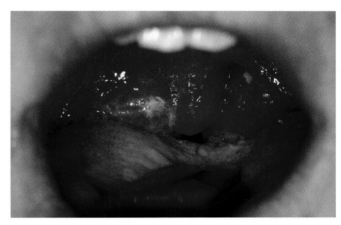

Figure 16.1 Acute tonsillitis.

associated with breathing difficulties, swallowing problems, the need to "clear the throat", also "bringing up" blood and/or the presence of a neck swelling or a lump.

The most common tissue involved in the inflammatory or infective process is the lymphoid tissue in the region, with the lateral oropharyngeal tissue (the tonsils) being the obvious and the easiest area to inspect with a tongue depressor and a good light source (Figure 16.1). Other areas where lymphoid tissue can become involved are the posterior tongue and the tissue located in the nasopharynx (the adenoids) collectively known as Waldeyer's ring. It should also be remembered that lymphoid tissue may be located in other areas of the pharynx superior to the vocal cords. Infective processes if left untreated may develop into a local collection of pus or an abscess. The most common is the peritonsillar abscess or quinsy, but other anatomical areas may also develop abscess particularly parapharyngeal and retropharyngeal areas, which if not recognised and treated early, may be life threatening.

Other tissues (nerves, muscles and cartilages) may be involved in inflammatory processes in the region, particularly with specific infections such as tuberculosis, syphilis, leprosy, AIDS and HIV, as well as with malignant disease including carcinoma and lymphoma.

Acute pharyngitis

Acute pharyngitis is defined by its most prominent symptom, i.e. acute onset sore throat, and has a primarily infectious aetiology.

While the term is used interchangeably with acute tonsillitis it is composed of a spectrum of conditions, most commonly viral in origin (40–60%), although bacteria may often be involved (5–30%), ranging from acute inflammation localised primarily to the tonsils to acute pharyngitis with generalised inflammation of the whole of the pharynx. Viral pathogens isolated include rhinoviruses, adenovirus, parainfluenza virus, coxsackie virus, Epstein–Barr virus (EBV; mononucleosis), cytomegalovirus (CMV) as well as human immunodeficiency virus (HIV). Group A beta-haemolytic streptococcus is the commonest cause of bacterial pharyngitis, but co-pathogens in children include *Staphylococcus aureus*, *Haemophilus influenzae*, *Branhamella catarrhalis* and *Bacteroides fragilis*. There is a short incubation period of 1–5 days and the great majority of individuals do not consult a doctor about their symptoms. Clinically differentiation of the pathogens of pharyngitis is rarely possible and there are no reliable clinical clues to identifying streptococcal infection. Frequently no pathogens are isolated on culture, making the value of this questionable.

Specific pharyngitis

Viral – infectious mononucleosis

Commonly known as glandular fever this is an acute, systemic viral infection presenting typically with sore throat and lymphadenopathy and usually due to the EBV, a human herpes virus. It is primarily a disease of young adults but can present in childhood and in older adults. Transmission is via saliva with an incubation period of between 5 and 7 days.

Initial presentation is with malaise, fatigue and headache for 4–5 days. The most common finding is tender cervical adenopathy, usually accompanied with a sore throat. The pharyngeal signs range from acute follicular tonsillitis indistinguishable from other causes of follicular tonsillitis, to a grey membrane lining the oropharynx, petechiae on the soft palate and sometimes a peritonsillar abscess, which can be bilateral. Systemic manifestations of EBV include hepatosplenomegaly, ascites and, more rarely, cranial nerve palsies, or a Guillain–Barré syndrome.

Diagnosis is made from the clinical picture, together with the finding of mononucleosis on the peripheral blood film. The monospot has a sensitivity of 86% and a specificity of 99%. False positive monospots can occur in healthy controls as well as in mumps, systemic lupus erythematosis and sarcoidosis. Treatment is symptomatic for mild to moderate cases. Ampicillin-based antibiotics should be avoided because of the certainty of producing a rubelliform rash. Acute airway obstruction secondary to EBV is an indication for steroid treatment.

Other viral diseases that may present in a similar manner include: cytomegalovirus, herpes simplex 1, herpes zoster, hand, foot and mouth disease and herpangina.

Other causes of specific pharyngitis

In the developing world and in vulnerable population groups, there are a number of conditions for which the clinician must be alert. These include HIV, TB, syphilis and other granulomatous disorders, inflammatory disorders of the oral cavity related to vasculitis, aphthous ulceration, lichen planus and Bechet's disease. Any non-healing lesion of the pharynx or oral cavity leads to the suspicion of neoplasia, both carcinoma and lymphoma, and early biopsy may be necessary for diagnosis.

HIV and AIDS

Oral lesions, especially pseudomembraneous and/or erythematous candidiasis and oral hairy leucoplakia, are highly suggestive of HIV infection in individuals of unknown HIV status. Widespread candidiasis in the oral cavity and oropharynx, with or without ulceration, should also suggest a possible association with HIV.

Lymphoid hyperplasia in the pharynx commonly involves all the tissues of Waldeyer's ring including adenoidal, palatine and lingual tonsils. Pharyngeal malignancy including Kaposi's sarcoma, non-Hodgkin's lymphoma and squamous cell carcinoma are all associated with patients with HIV/AIDS.

Tuberculosis

The pharynx is not a common site for the clinical manifestation of tuberculosis. It is the site of primary infection almost always in children and results in an asymptomatic primary focus in the pharynx (usually tonsil or adenoid) with cervical lymphadenopathy. In adults the pharynx may be involved in patients with widespread miliary tuberculosis. Pharyngeal tuberculosis is treated as the pulmonary disease with triple therapy.

Syphilis

This is an infection by the spirochaete *Treponema pallidum* and apart from the congenital form, is acquired by sexual intercourse. In secondary syphilis the pharynx and soft palate display hyperaemia and inflammation and there may be lesions which have been described as mucous patches or "snail track" ulcers. The lesions are more commonly seen in the oral cavity than in the oropharynx. These lesions may last for several weeks. Confirmation of the disease is by testing for the specific antibody TPI and is 100% specific in patients with established secondary and tertiary syphilis. Penicillin is the treatment of choice with 2.4 mega units intramuscular in single or divided doses, being the standard for primary and secondary syphilis.

Diphtheria

Corynebacterium diphtheria is the pathogen which leads to diphtheria. Uncommon in the Western World because of widespread immunisation in children but is on the increase in the non-immunised patients.

Patients complain of severe sore throat, low-grade fever and cervical adenopathy. Sometimes accompanied by malaise, headache and nausea. Significant is the sweet fetor from the mouth. Tonsillar infection leads to acute pharyngitis characterised by a grey, velvety firm adherent pseudomembranes covering the tonsils (Figure 16.2). When the membrane is wiped off the underlying surface bleeds easily. Systemic effect of the toxins can lead to myocarditis, nephritis and encephalitis.

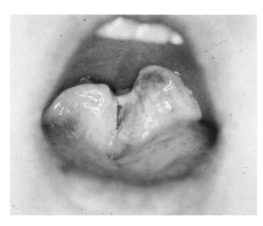

Figure 16.2 Diphtheria tonsillitis.

Diagnosis is made by suspicion, and obtaining a smear and culture (Krebs–Loeffler medium) tests. Treatment of diphtheria should start immediately and antitoxin should be given within the first 48 h of onset without confirmation of the result of the throat swab. Allergic testing to ensure no allergy against horse serum should be done before injection. Antibiotics are also required to treat the local symptoms. Patients need to be isolated for 2–4 days after adequate therapy to prevent cross infection.

Clinical signs of pharyngitis

Clinical signs and the appearance of the throat may vary but are not a reliable indicator of the precise nature of the infection (Box 16.1).

Box 16.1 **Clinical signs of pharyngitis**

- Pain in the throat and difficulty in swallowing
- Pain radiating to the ears
- Variable erythema of the pharynx and the tonsils are swollen and may be coated
- Pyrexia
- Swollen lymph nodes under the jaw and in the neck may occur

---

Treatment

Many patients can be treated with simple analgesia, such as paracetamol or a non-steroidal anti-inflammatory drug, in combination if required. Aspirin should be avoided in children because of the risk of Reye's syndrome. Benzydamine (Difflam) gargles may also be helpful. The routine use of an antibiotic is illogical, unnecessary and potentially hazardous as most sore throats are viral and there is a favourable outcome in most patients, with resolution within 2–3 days. However, if the sore throat is very severe or shows no sign of improvement after 2–3 days, antibiotic therapy should not be withheld as bacterial super-infection may have occurred or more serious complications may be developing.

Recurrent sore throat

The reason for sore throat occurring recurrently is not fully understood, but is likely to be related to fluctuating immunity as much to pathology within the tonsils themselves, or to the efficacy of any therapy employed. The evidence is now strong that a significant majority of a cohort of sufferers in the paediatric age group show improvement over 3 years with most having only minor episodes thereafter. Cohorts of children treated conservatively show similar levels of symptoms to those treated by tonsillectomy after 3 years, but there are individual cases that continue to have severe recurrent episodes resulting in significant morbidity. There is also a group of adults, typically in the teens or early 20s, who suffer recurrent or chronic sore throat symptoms with disabling morbidity from time to time. This problem sems to diminish after the age of 30 years.

Indications for tonsillectomy

By definition, tonsillitis cannot occur after tonsillectomy (unless some tonsillar remnants are present). It is therefore important in considering tonsillectomy that the diagnosis of tonsil pathology is as certain as possible. The indications for tonsillectomy have become more stringent recently as a better understanding of the risk–benefit analysis has developed. Following the recent revision of the SIGN Guideline on sore throat, tonsillectomy should now be considered if the criteria in Box 16.2 are met.

Box 16.2 **Indications for tonsillectomy**

- Sore throat is due to tonsillitis
- The episodes of sore throat are disabling and prevent normal activity
- Seven or more well-documented, clinically significant and adequately treated episodes in the preceding year
- Five or more such episodes in each of the preceding 2 years
- Three or more such episodes in each of the preceding 3 years

---

The benefits must be balanced against the small but significant risk of complications, particularly haemorrhage (which has an incidence of 2–8% in one national audit) and because the operation itself carries morbidity, usually lasting for around 2 weeks, but which is at least predictable. Management of this includes adequate analgesia, anti-emetics when required and attention to nutrition, oral hygiene and hydration.

Complications of sore throat

Following streptococcal infection, complications may occur and rarely in the developed world include rheumatic fever (0.3% of cases untreated cases) and glomerulonephritis. Septic complications are much commoner after both viral and bacterial tonsillitis as bacterial superinfection may occur following an initial viral infection and may result in serious and occasionally life threatening illness.

Quinsy

Peritonsillar abscess (quinsy) is a collection of pus between the fibrous capsule of the tonsil and the superior constrictor muscle of the pharynx. The upper pole is the most frequent location. It is usually a complication of acute tonsillitis, occurs at any age, but is most often seen in young adults between 20 and 40 years. The bacteriology of a quinsy when cultured often grows anaerobic organisms as well as the usual beta-haemolytic streptococcal infection.

Clinically the history is progressive, usually unilateral, sore throat over 3 or 4 days, pain on swallowing (odynophagia), dysphagia for solids and eventually liquids, drooling of saliva, trismus, ipsilateral ear pain and headache associated with fever, lethargy and ipsilateral lymphadenopathy. The patient usually develops a "plummy voice" secondary to the oropharyngeal swelling. There is limited opening of the mouth, with the tonsil displaced medially by the bulging in the region of the superior pole of the tonsil and enlarged tender lymph nodes in the upper jugulodigastric area of the neck. The differential diagnosis includes infectious, inflammatory, vascular and neoplastic pathologies (Box 16.3).

> Box 16.3 **Differential diagnosis of quinsy**
>
> - **Infectious**: peritonsillar cellulitis, parapharyngeal abscess, upper molar dental abscess, and infectious mononucleosis.
> - **Inflammatory**: Kawasaki disease (rare)
> - **Vascular**: post-traumatic internal carotid pseudo-aneurysm (rare)
> - **Malignant neoplasm**: squamous cell carcinoma, lymphoma, sarcoma, metastatic disease, minor salivary gland tumour.
> - **Benign neoplasm**: deep lobe parotid lesions (rare)

Confirmation of the presence of pus on needle aspiration is diagnostic, but if there is doubt, or the patient is very ill and there is difficulty evaluating the anatomical region, then imaging is indicated prior to any surgical intervention. The use of ultrasound or CT scan is able to differentiate severe cellulitis from abscess in most cases.

Treatment of quinsy

Most patients diagnosed with a quinsy will be admitted to hospital for intravenous fluids and antibiotics until acceptable swallowing has recovered. Benzylpenicillin intravenously will cover the majority of the anaerobes as well as the streptococcal infection and is the treatment of choice, but metronidazole may also be added. Patients allergic to penicillin should be treated with erythromycin. The use of steroids in addition has been shown to speed recovery, reducing throat pain, time in hospital, fever and trismus, with no increase in complications. The presence of a pointing abscess, clinical deterioration, failure to respond to intravenous antibiotic and evidence of an abscess on imaging, would all be reasonable indications for drainage either by needle aspiration or using a conventional guarded quinsy knife.

Abscess tonsillectomy has been advocated in some clinical environments, but has not been routine in the UK. Good results and minimal morbidity are reported with no increase in perioperative, primary or secondary haemorrhage and the additional advantage of avoiding recurrence and the need for elective delayed tonsillectomy.

Complications of quinsy

Deep neck space abscess and mediastinitis have been described. Mediastinitis has a significant mortality even when treated aggressively with powerful antibiotics. Predisposing factors include immune suppression related to such causes as diabetes, steroid therapy, HIV and drug dependency.

Parapharyngeal abscess

The parapharyngeal space is a potential space located on either side of the upper pharynx, from the nasopharynx to the oropharynx. Infection can spread to the parapharyngeal space from any of the other deep neck spaces including peritonsillar, retropharyngeal and submandibular space. The most common source of infection is tonsil and dental sepsis.

Bacteriology of deep neck space infections seems to be changing with increasing numbers of cases due to gram-negative aerobic organisms, which do not respond to first-line penicillin treatment and thus may be contributing to the significant mortality seen in some parts of the world. Organisms such as *Klebsiella pneumonia* and *Streptcoccus viridians* are commonly grown.

Presentation and examination are very similar to peritonsillar abscess except that the maximum swelling in the pharynx is more inferiorly placed and behind the tonsil, with less oedema of the palate. Not infrequently, a firm but fluctuant swelling rather than lymphadenopathy can be felt in the upper neck. The differential diagnosis is similar to peritonsillar abscess and if the diagnosis is suspected, then a CT scan of the head (Figure 16.3), neck and chest is advisable while treatment is commenced. Treatment is in

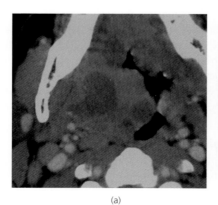
(a)

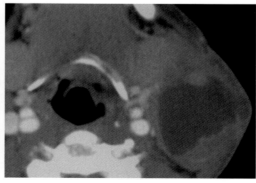
(b)

Figure 16.3 (a) Tonsillar and parapharyngeal abscess; (b) large neck abscess secondary to tonsillitis.

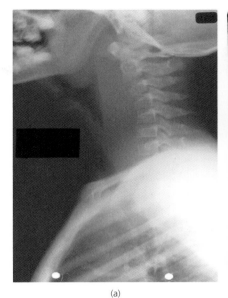 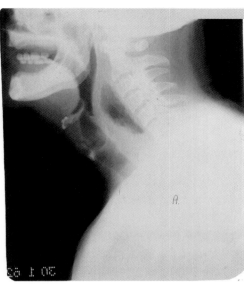

Figure 16.4 (a) Lateral soft tissue of neck X-ray showing an abscess widening of the retropharyngeal space; (b) cavitation of a retropharyngeal abscess.

(a)   (b)

hospital, with particular attention to the elective management of the airway either by intubation or, if necessary, tracheostomy. Surgical drainage may be necessary if the clinical condition does not respond rapidly to intravenous antibiotics with or without steroids and if a collection is demonstrated on imaging.

Retropharyngeal abscess

Retropharyngeal abscess most commonly occurs in children under 6 years old, with a peak incidence between 3 and 5 years. It is due to suppurating retropharyngeal lymph nodes following an upper respiratory tract infection. The most common organism is *Streptococcus viridans* with or without gram-negative organisms. Rarely, it may occur following foreign body penetration such as a fishbone or an abscess of the cervical spine usually associated with tuberculosis.

Clinical features

The typical case is a young child with a history of an upper respiratory tract infection with additional features of a stiff neck, or holding the neck to one side and associated with fever, irritability, dysphagia and noisy breathing with, on examination, the posterior pharyngeal wall bulging forward. This diagnosis can be

overlooked and should be considered in children with fever and irritability. A lateral soft tissue X-ray of neck may assist diagnosis (Figure 16.4). The possibility of epiglottitis, now rare in children following immunisation against *Haemophilus influenzi*, should be borne in mind. Adults may have few symptoms, with severe pain on swallowing presenting at a relatively late stage, and the differential diagnosis may include nasopharyngeal cancer, lipomas, and carotid aneurysm. Investigation is by CT scan, followed by surgical drainage which may be needle aspiration or open drainage followed by intravenous antibiotics. Extreme care is necessary during intubation in these cases because of the danger of abscess rupture and aspiration of pus.

Further reading

Burton MJ, Glasziou PP. Tonsillectomy or adeno-tonsillectomy versus non-surgical treatment for chronic/recurrent acute tonsillitis. *Cochrane Database Syst Rev* 2009;Issue 1:CD001802. doi: 10.1002/14651858 .CD001802.pub2

Spinks A, Glasziou PP, Del Mar CB. Antibiotics for sore throat. *Cochrane Database Syst Rev* 2006;Issue 4:CD000023.

SIGN Guideline 117. Management of sore throat and indications for tonsillectomy. www.sign.ac.uk/guidelines/fulltext/117/index.html

CHAPTER 17

Hoarseness and Voice Disorders

Mered Harries

Brighton and Sussex University Hospitals, Brighton, UK

OVERVIEW

- Any patient who is hoarse for longer than 3 weeks needs an urgent chest X-ray, and if negative an ENT referral for a laryngoscopy
- Any patient with "red flag" symptoms should be referred urgently
- Understanding the anatomy and physiology of the larynx allows the clinician to make an accurate provisional diagnosis from the history and listening to the patient's voice
- Histologically proven laryngeal cancer in an early stage is likely to be cured
- Assessment in the ENT clinic ideally involves a multidisciplinary approach with a speech and language therapist and laryngologist

What is voice?

There are three essential components to voice production:

1 An air source – the lungs
2 A vibrating source – the vocal cords
3 A resonating chamber – the volume between the vocal cords and the openings of the lips and nostrils – this space is termed the **vocal tract.**

A problem located with any of the three listed above can affect voice – for example if you pinch your nose the voice assumes a nasal quality – but this chapter will concentrate on disorders of the larynx and the vocal cords.

The human voice – unique!

In most animals the larynx lies either above or at the level of the palate (or its equivalent). In some cases this allows constant stimulation of the olfactory organs which are much more sensitive than in the human and necessary for survival, but more importantly it separates the feeding passages from the airway. The human is

ABC of Ear, Nose and Throat, Sixth Edition.
Edited by Harold Ludman and Patrick J. Bradley.
© 2013 John Wiley & Sons, Ltd. Published 2013 by John Wiley & Sons, Ltd.

unique in that the larynx descends down to the level of the sixth cervical vertebra which increases the volume of the vocal tract and contributes to the complexity of the human voice. As a result of this lower position the primary function of the larynx is to protect the distal tracheobronchial tree and prevent any aspiration and voice production is very much secondary to this. The third function of the larynx is to provide a closed glottis so that the diaphragm can be splinted for lifting and/or straining (Box 17.1).

Box 17.1 **Functions of the larynx**

- Protection of the distal tracheobronchial tree
- Production of voice
- Closed glottis on straining or lifting to give support to the diaphragm

Anatomy of the larynx

There are three divisions (Figure 17.1):

1 *Supraglottis* – above the vocal cords and including the epiglottis and false cords
2 *Glottis* – the true vocal cords, the vibrating parts of which are the membranous vocal folds
3 *Subglottis* – extends from the vocal cords to the start of the trachea at the lower border of the cricoid cartilage. It is the narrowest part of the airways and oedema here causes stridor – especially in children where 1mm of swelling of the mucosal lining can reduce the airway by 25% or more. The subglottis is also the area where any trauma with an anaesthetic tube can cause permanent stenosis which may require a tracheostomy.

Embryology

The larynx is the perfect organ to demonstrate the importance of embryology and how easy it is to remember its anatomy and nerve supply. The supraglottis comes from the IVth branchial arch (nerve supply: superior laryngeal nerve) – the Vth branchial arch disappears in the human – the subglottis from the VIth branchial arch (nerve supply: recurrent laryngeal nerve). The glottis lies between these and as a result has very poor lymphatic

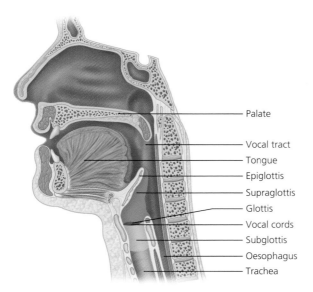

Figure 17.1 Cross section showing the vocal tract and subdivisions of the larynx.

Palate
Vocal tract
Tongue
Epiglottis
Supraglottis
Glottis
Vocal cords
Subglottis
Oesophagus
Trachea

drainage – inflammation can give very swollen vocal cords but conversely any glottic tumour has a good prognosis as its lymphatic spread is poor – a T1 carcinoma of the glottis has a 95% cure rate either with radiotherapy or laser resection.

Remember that the laryngeal nerves lie in close proximity to the thyroid gland and can be damaged at surgery. It is also worth remembering that the recurrent laryngeal nerve on the left passes down into the chest so that one of the presenting signs of a bronchial tumour may be hoarseness.

Vocal cords in normal voice

The vocal cords open (abduct) to allow breathing and close (adduct) during voice production (Figure 17.2).

As air passes up from the lungs it causes the membranous parts of the vocal cords (vocal folds) to vibrate. The vocal folds vibrate 100 times per second in the male and almost double this in the female – this gives the female voice a higher pitch but may also explain the predominance of vocal pathology in females. To vibrate at this rate, the vocal folds need to be well lubricated – consider

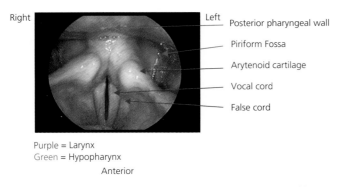

Right
Left
Posterior pharyngeal wall
Piriform Fossa
Arytenoid cartilage
Vocal cord
False cord

Purple = Larynx
Green = Hypopharynx
Anterior

Figure 17.2 The ''normal anatomy'' of the larynx and hypopharynx (the vocal cords are in their resting position).

trying to blow a raspberry with dry versus moist lips. The dryness associated with any inflammation will affect vibration hence the importance of steam inhalations and good hydration in these situations, especially in singers.

Changes in the vocal folds can be considered in four subgroups:

1 Increase in mass lowers the pitch of the voice
2 Poor closure of the two vocal folds gives a breathy and weak voice
3 Increase in stiffness leads to poor vibration and a rough, harsh voice
4 Any lesion on the free edge of the fold gives an irregular voice with pitch breaks.

Listening to the quality of the voice and combining this with a good history can often give a very good idea of the likely pathology and although any patient with hoarseness for more than 6 weeks should be referred for examination of their larynx, it can help identify who needs to be seen urgently.

Laryngeal examination

There have been major technological advancements in laryngeal examination and voice assessment over the past 15 years. The larynx can be viewed with a flexible endoscope inserted via the nose (Figure 17.3) or with a rigid angled telescope via the mouth (Figure 17.4). Both give excellent views, especially the distal chip scopes. The flexible scope has the advantage of showing not only structure but also giving a dynamic assessment of how the vocal cords are being used to produce voice whereas the rigid scopes give excellent magnification and can be used for stroboscopy.

The human eye can only discern five images per second and any signal faster than this is perceived as a blur – remember flicking through cartoon books as a child. The vocal folds are vibrating at

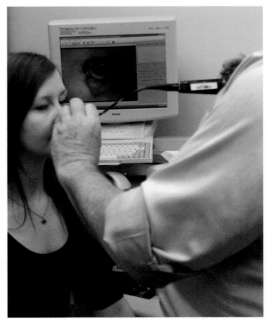

Figure 17.3 Examination of the larynx using a video flexible nasendoscope.

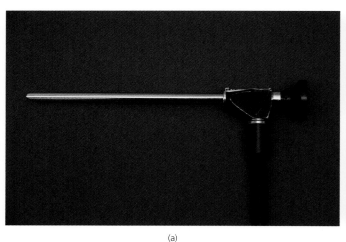
(a)

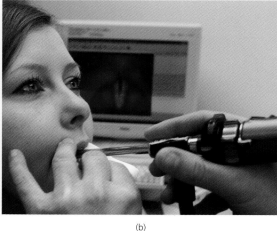
(b)

Figure 17.4 (a) A 90° rigid laryngoscope; (b) its application to view the larynx transorally with a picture on the video monitor.

speeds greater than 100 times per second so observation with white light will only show a blurred edge. By adjusting the light shutter speed to a rate slightly different to the rate of vocal fold vibration, we are able to produce a montage of apparent slow-motion vocal fold vibration. This is the principle of stroboscopy. The periodic vibration of the vocal folds is also termed the mucosal wave and abnormalities such as scarring and submucosal cysts can be picked up with stroboscopy but appear normal on white light examination. It is now recommended that any professional voice user with a voice disorder should ideally be seen in a voice clinic with stroboscopy and other voice assessment tools such as acoustic analysis.

Aetiology of voice disorders

These can be divided into four basic categories although there can be considerable overlap:

1 Neoplastic
2 Inflammatory
3 Neuromuscular
4 Technical (also termed muscle tension or misuse).

Aetiologies of hoarseness

These are outlined in Table 17.1.

What to ask for in the history?

Voice problems are not uncommon so it is important to be able to identify potentially serious cases from the history and listening to the patients' voice. Specific questions to ask are shown in Box 17.2.

Box 17.2 **Specific questions to ask when taking a history**

Timing

- Acute/chronic in onset: associated with URTI?
- Constant or intermittent?
- Duration?
- Precipitating factors: voice use/abuse (shouting, screaming, Karaoke)?
- Occupation: how long in post? How much voice use?
- Relieving factors: voice rest?

Associated symptoms

- Dysphagia (difficulty swallowing)
- Odynophagia (painful swallowing)
- Otalgia (referred pain to the ear)
- Haemoptysis
- Weight loss
- Dyspnoea
- Stridor

Table 17.1 Aetiologies of hoarseness.

Neoplastic/structural	Inflammatory	Neuromuscular	Muscle tension/technical
Benign	**Infective**	**Hypofunctional**	Vocal strain/technique
Cysts	Bacterial	Parkinson's	Excess demands /occupation
Polyps	Fungal	Myasthenia gravis	Psychogenic
Scarring	Viral	Bulbar palsy	Anxiety
Haemorrhage	**Non-infective**	**Hyperfunctional**	Stress
Presbylaryngeal (bowing)	Allergy	Chorea	Postural strain
Malignant	Reflux	Spasmodic dysphonia	
Carcinoma	Smoking		
Nodules	Autoimmune		
Reinke's Oedema	Traumatic (including voice abuse)		

Social factors

- Smoking: quantity and duration
- Alcohol
- Dietary habits: laryngopharyngeal reflux?
- Caffeine and fluid intake

Associated medical conditions

- Asthma: ALL patients using inhalers should be instructed to not only rinse out the mouth but also to gargle after using ANY inhaler. Steroids can predispose to candida but all inhalers can have a drying irritation effect on vocal fold vibration
- Cardiovascular medications can affect the larynx indirectly due to dryness and irritation especially some beta-blockers
- Neuromuscular conditions such as Parkinson's disease, myasthenia gravis and motor neurone disease

Psychological and psychiatric conditions

- Anxiety
- Stress
- Depression

Dangerous "red flag" symptoms suggest urgent referral to the ENT department:

S – Smoker, Stridor
C – Constant/persistent hoarseness, Coughing up blood
A – Acute onset *not* related to URTI, Alcohol
L – Loss of weight
D – Dyspnoea, Dysphagia.

Treatments

These are in three main areas:

Voice therapy – Includes vocal hygiene advice on lubrication, hydration and avoidance of irritants such as smoking and caffeine. Technical advice as well as correction of posture to reduce muscle tension.
Medical therapy – Includes appropriate use of antibiotics, antifungals, antireflux medications including dietary advice and Botulinum toxin injections for spasmodic dysphonia.
Surgical therapy – Includes endolaryngeal surgery with laser and laryngeal framework surgery via open approach though the neck.

The following case presentations highlight the importance of history and listening to the voice of the patient to obtain a diagnosis and identify patients that need urgent referral.

Read the history and look at the image before reading the diagnosis.

Case 1

Betty Belt (24) is a primary school teacher and a budding actress. She is active in the local dramatic society and has recently successfully auditioned for the role of Maria in the forthcoming production of the Sound of Music. She has noticed a gradual onset of voice

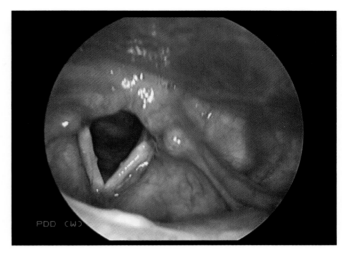

Figure 17.5 Bilateral swellings on the vocal cords which prevent full closure.

change, worse at the end of the day and especially bad after a night out socialising. She is a non-smoker, consumes little alcohol, but is particularly partial to a kipper on a Saturday morning. Her voice is harsh and breathy with obvious pitch breaks

What's relevant?

Voice use – both speaking and singing.
Young – only in post for a year.
Gradual onset
Non-smoker
Breathy – poor closure
Harsh – edge of vocal fold not smooth
Pitch breaks – edge of vocal fold not smooth
Laryngoscopic – Figure 17.5.
Diagnosis – vocal nodules.
Treatment – speech therapy.

The kipper is not relevant – it is in fact a red herring!

Case 2

Alf Player is a 62-year-old smoker – 20 a day for over 40 years – who works in the building trade. He lives alone and consumes two bottles of whisky a week. He presents with a 3-month history of sudden onset change in voice following a viral illness. His voice is of normal pitch but is constantly weak and breathy and tires towards the end of the day. No dyspnoea, but has noticed that he does cough if he drinks quickly and has had one episode of haemoptysis.

What's relevant?

Smoking – heavy
Occupation – dust, asbestos exposure?
Acute onset, short duration, constant
Alcohol intake – heavy
Breathy/weak – poor closure
Aspiration – incompetent larynx.
Haemoptysis – ?source
Laryngoscopic – Figure 17.6.

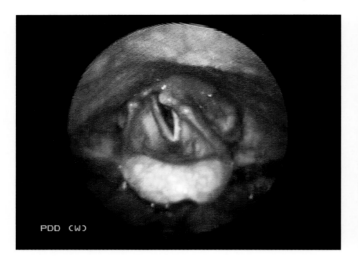

Figure 17.6 The left vocal cord is bowed, shortened and not abducted compared to the right cord.

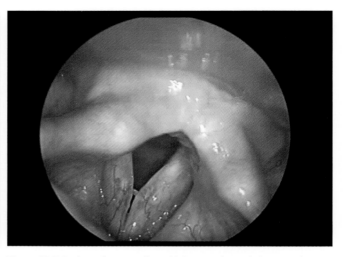

Figure 17.7 Both cords are swollen with increased vascularity secondary to inflammation. There is a band of sticky mucus crossing from one cord to the other – termed "mucous bridging", which reflects poor hydration and lubrication.

Diagnosis – Left vocal cord paralysis probably secondary to lung cancer. A CT chest would confirm this.

Treatment – Radiotherapy to the advanced bronchial tumour and an injection to bulk/medialise the left vocal cord to allow the cords to meet.

Case 3

Edna Belch is a 42-year-old female publican. She has smoked 20 cigarettes a day for over 20 years and enjoys life to the full. She is a member of the pub's darts team and enjoys a curry at least twice a week. She takes a range of medications including Gaviscon. She has noticed that her voice has become deeper over the last 9 months and was very upset when she was recently mistaken for a man on the phone during a dating agency interview.

What's relevant?

Female with voice use and abuse
Smoker
Laryngopharyngeal reflux
Lower pitch – mass increased
Gradual onset – persistent voice change.
Laryngoscopic – Figure 17.7.

Diagnosis – Gross oedema of the vocal folds (Reinke's oedema).

Treatment – Remove irritants, treat reflux, improve vocal hygiene and speech therapy. Surgery to trim and reduce the vibrating mass of the vocal folds can be considered after a period of an aggressive conservative approach.

Case 4

James Screech is a well known lead singer in a famous Rock band. As he walked onto the stage in Hammersmith he yelled at the audience and felt a sharp pain at the level of the larynx. He has unable to finish the performance and now (2 weeks later) has a rough, deep voice with numerous pitch breaks. He cannot sing and remarkably is a non-smoker. He denies any drug abuse and his alcohol intake is moderate not exceeding the weekly recommendations.

What's relevant?

Acute onset associated with voice abuse
Rough voice and pitch breaks – irregular contact of vocal folds
Non-smoker
Laryngoscopic – Figure 17.8.

Diagnosis – Vocal fold haemorrhagic polyp.

Treatment – Surgical excision via microlaryngoscopy and laser. The carbon dioxide laser has excellent precision and haemostatic properties and would be used for most vascular laryngeal lesions. To minimise likely recurrence, advice and voice coaching is advised pre- and post-operatively by a speech and language therapist.

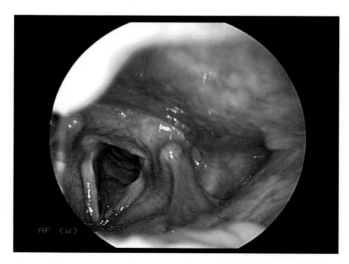

Figure 17.8 Large red swelling on the left vocal cord.

Conclusions

A thorough understanding of the anatomy and physiology of the larynx helps clinicians diagnose voice disorders. Although every patient with hoarseness should be referred to the ENT department for a laryngoscopy, taking a relevant history and listening to the voice can assist in prioritising patients with possible serious conditions. Although by no means comprehensive, the case histories highlight the different aetiologies of hoarseness and the different management strategies available.

Further reading

Benninger M, Murry M. *The Performer's Voice*. Pleural Publishing Inc., 2006.
Fried M, Fertilo AA. *The Larynx*. Pleural Publishing Inc., 2009.

CHAPTER 18

Airway Obstruction and Stridor

Vinidh Paleri[1] and Patrick J. Bradley[2]

[1]Newcastle upon Tyne Hospitals, Newcastle, UK
[2]Nottingham University Hospitals, Queen's Medical Centre Campus, Nottingham, UK

OVERVIEW

- Airway obstruction may present as an emergency, requires a high index of suspicion to prevent a catastrophe, and should prompt immediate hospitalisation
- Stridor is caused by turbulent flow of air through a partially obstructed segment of the respiratory tract and can be diagnosed on the phase it manifests in the respiratory cycle
- Acute sudden onset of stridor, in an apyrexial and previously normal person, should arouse suspicion that a foreign body has been aspirated
- In the absence of any definitive precipitating cause and relevant history, acute and chronic stridor in adults should be considered to be neoplastic until proven otherwise

---

Of all emergencies seen in otolaryngologic practice, diagnosing and managing airway obstruction is one of the most complex, needing multiprofessional input and an experienced team to achieve good outcomes. The upper airway can be obstructed by a range of disease processes, from pathology in the anterior nasal cavity to the lower airways. Problems associated with breathing usually present as nasal obstruction, stertor and stridor. Nasal diseases are discussed elsewhere and this chapter will focus on pathology in the larynx, pharynx and trachea that causes airway obstruction.

Pathophysiology

Breathing is under involuntary control and is mediated by the respiratory centre in the brainstem. The vocal cords abduct during inspiration and with the negative pressure caused by diaphragmatic contraction and expansion of the lungs, air is drawn into the lungs. The recurrent laryngeal branches of the vagus nerves control vocal cord movement, with a complex arrangement of intrinsic muscles in the larynx providing fine control. The cricoid cartilage is the only complete ring in the respiratory tract, and surrounds the subglottic region. Thus, any airway oedema compromises the lumen, and even a minimal reduction in the airway can cause dramatic compromise of the airflow. Thus, 1 mm of mucosal oedema reduces the cross-sectional area by more than 40%.

Stridor is a harsh, vibratory noise caused by turbulent flow of air through a partially obstructed segment of the respiratory tract. This should be differentiated from **stertor**, where the noise is caused by vibration of the pharyngeal structures, such as the soft palate, during sleep and leads to a lower-pitched noise. Respiratory distress may not be a feature where a chronic, non-progressive lesion causes stridor and the patient has adapted well. Stridor can be present during the inspiratory or the expiratory phase or be biphasic; this can inform the site of obstruction (Box 18.1).

Box 18.1 **Types of stridor**

- **Inspiratory**: supraglottic and glottic obstruction
- **Expiratory**: low tracheal obstruction
- **Biphasic**: glottic and subglottic obstruction

Stridor in children

Evaluation

A careful history provides useful pointers to the diagnosis (Box 18.2). A previously well child presenting with acute onset stridor should arouse suspicions of foreign body aspiration. A preceding upper respiratory tract infection (URTI) indicates croup or bacterial tracheitis. Epiglottitis (supraglottitis) typically presents as rapid onset fever, dysphagia and drooling in children aged between 2 and 7 years.

Box 18.2 **Historical information**

- Age of onset
- Duration/phase of stridor
- Worsening/improvement of stridor since onset
- Precipitating causes
- Failure to gain weight
- Breath-holding spells
- Fever
- Feeding /swallowing problems
- Hoarse/muffled voice
- Intubation in the past
- Cough/chest infections

ABC of Ear, Nose and Throat, Sixth Edition.
Edited by Harold Ludman and Patrick J. Bradley.
© 2013 John Wiley & Sons, Ltd. Published 2013 by John Wiley & Sons, Ltd.

The child with acute stridor is ideally assessed in a setting where instrumentation and experienced personnel are available for emergency intervention to secure and stabilise the airway. The areas that clinical assessment should cover are shown in Box 18.3. Respiratory rate and level of consciousness are the most important indicators of severity of obstruction. Increasing intensity of the sound is not an indicator of the severity, as in severe obstruction the airflow is significantly diminished and thus no stridor may be heard. Measures should be taken not distress the child further for fear of precipitating an acute obstruction. This includes keeping the parent or carer at all times with the child, until the airway is secure. With increasing hypoxia and carbon dioxide retention, the child can become drowsy and unresponsive.

Box 18.3 **Clinical evaluation**

- Respiratory rate
- Cyanosis
- Apnoeic spells
- Use of accessory muscles
- Intercostal/sternal retraction
- Nasal flaring
- Timing/severity of stridor
- Hoarseness
- Temperature/toxicity
- Level of consciousness
- ENT examination in controlled setting

A working diagnosis of the cause of obstruction can be made in the majority of cases before direct examination of the airway (Figure 18.1). Most of these conditions are in the evolving phase when initially seen, and if observation only is planned, this is best done in an intensive care or high-dependency setting where rapid intervention is possible if the patient deteriorates.

Congenital structural lesions rarely present in the acute setting. For children with chronic stridor a diagnostic laryngotracheoscopy will be required in the majority of patients, unless the condition is mild and readily diagnosed on clinical examination alone. In the cooperative child with no evidence of hypoxia, flexible laryngoscopy in the clinic can be very informative. Surgical treatment is usually necessary for chronic obstruction that doesn't respond to conservative treatment.

Acute stridor

Retropharyngeal and peritonsillar abscesses

Drooling, painful swallowing and systemic upset are usually seen at presentation, usually with a preceding URTI. Retropharyngeal abscesses in the lower pharynx can cause laryngeal oedema and stridor. Neck stiffness and torticollis, if present, can help differentiate this condition from supraglottitis. Once suspected, imaging is recommended to confirm the diagnosis and identify the extent of the abscess collection (Figure 18.2). Peritonsillar abscesses are associated with trismus and more likely to present with stertor and do not need imaging. Urgent drainage is required for both conditions.

Supraglottitis

Haemophilus influenzae type B is the usual infective agent, although the incidence has significantly decreased with HiB vaccination. Children between the ages of 2 and 7 years of age are affected, with a peak incidence in 3-year-olds. The disease typically presents with

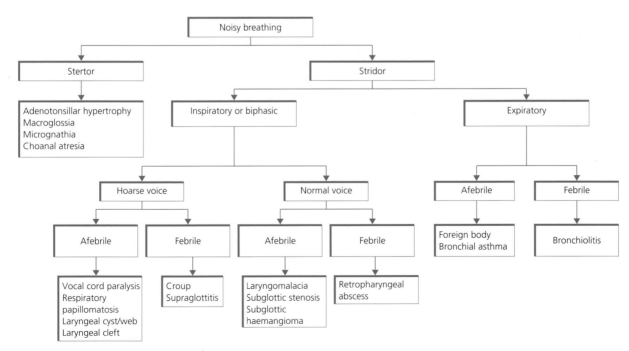

Figure 18.1 Differential diagnosis of stridor in children.

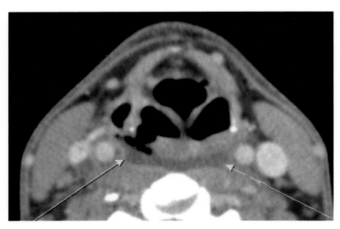

Figure 18.2 CT image of a retropharyngeal abscess showing an abscess cavity (arrowed) and generalised soft tissue swelling.

a rapid onset of high fever, toxicity, agitation, stridor, dyspnoea, muffled voice and painful swallowing. Examination will reveal a child seated and leaning forward with the mouth open and drooling. If supraglottitis is suspected, no further examination is recommended outside of a controlled setting. In acute supraglottitis, the risk of complete obstruction is high and the airway has to be secured. Endotracheal intubation is the method of choice as the supraglottic swelling is usually reversible in a few days, unless complications occur. An oedematous, cherry-red epiglottis with inflammation of the surrounding supraglottis is seen on direct laryngoscopy (Figure 18.3). Intravenous antibiotics are required.

Laryngotracheobronchitis

The most common cause of acute stridor in childhood is laryngotracheobronchitis or croup. Parainfluenza virus is the most common causative agent, with influenza virus types A or B, respiratory syncytial virus and rhinoviruses also being implicated. Children between the ages of 6 months and 3 years are affected, with a peak incidence in the second year of life. A history of preceding upper respiratory tract infection is usually present. Symptoms include low-grade fever, barking cough, inspiratory stridor and hoarseness. These are characteristically worse at night and are aggravated by agitation and crying. If the diagnosis is clear, no endoscopy is needed. Nebulised adrenaline with intravenous steroids is recommended in croup. Severe cases may need intubation and ventilation.

Chronic stridor

Gastro-oesophageal reflux is a very common problem in children with chronic stridor that has been noted in up to 80% of patients. This is partly caused by the strong thoraco-abdominal pressure gradient seen in airway obstruction. While reflux can make an existing condition, such as laryngomalacia, worse, an aetiologic role in conditions such as subglottic stenosis has been proposed. There is no consensus on routine treatment of reflux in these patients.

Laryngomalacia

This condition accounts for 75% of all causes of stridor in infants. **Weakness and laxity** of the supraglottic structures leads to prolapse of the supraglottis during inspiration, causing airway compromise (Figures 18.4 and 18.5). This presents as inspiratory or variable stridor between the fourth and sixth weeks of life. Stridor is typically worsened by crying and feeding and relieved when in the prone position. This is a self-limiting condition and surgery is not indicated unless the added work of breathing causes failure to thrive and feeding problems. Supraglottoplasty involves

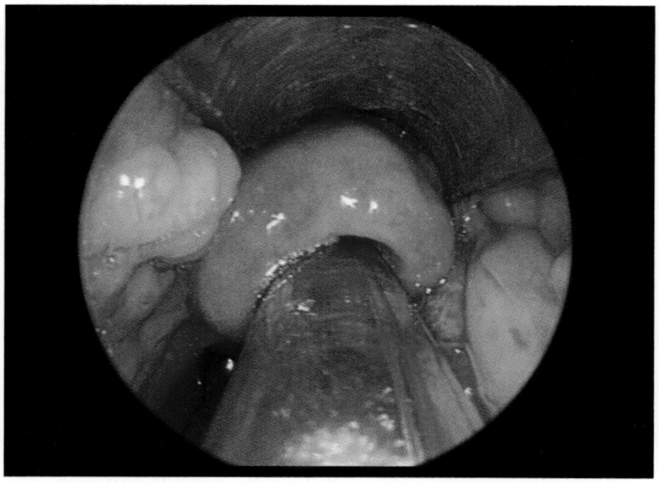

Figure 18.3 Laryngoscopic view of oedematous and red epiglottis, with generalised oedema of supraglottic.

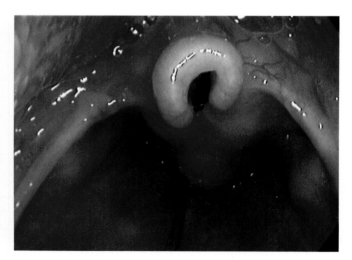

Figure 18.4 Laryngomalacia showing open airway during expiration. (Courtesy of Dr H. Kubba)

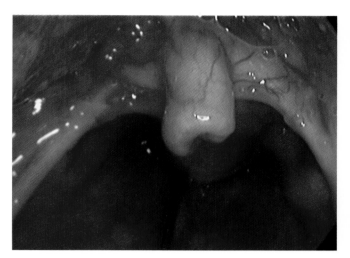

Figure 18.5 Laryngomalacia showing epiglottis collapse during inspiration. (Courtesy Dr H. Kubba)

dividing the shortened aryepiglottic folds and reducing supraglottic collapse.

Subglottic stenosis

This entity can be congenital or iatrogenic in origin, the latter secondary to prolonged intubation and ventilation (Figure 18.6). Presenting symptoms include inspiratory or biphasic stridor, usually in the first year of life. Iatrogenic stenosis should be suspected in the setting of an inability to wean the child off the

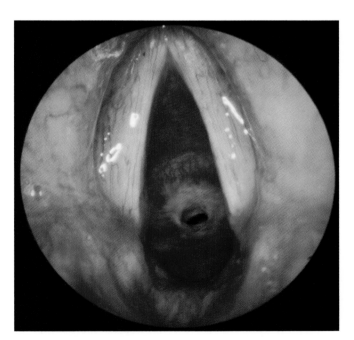

Figure 18.6 Severe congenital subglottic stenosis. (Courtesy of Dr T McGill, Boston, USA)

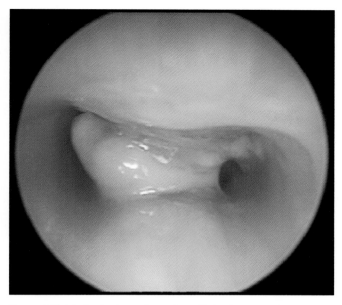

Figure 18.7 Intratracheal granuloma above the tracheostomy site, preventing weening off a ventilator. (Courtesy of Dr T. McGill, Boston, USA)

ventilator or stridor presenting after extubation (Figure 18.7). Milder stenoses can be observed and with laryngeal growth, the narrowing may not cause obstruction. Surgical reconstruction may be required for the severe ones.

Vocal cord paralysis

Presentation is typically within the first month of life. Stridor, cyanosis, apnoea and feeding problems are seen. Concomitant neurologic disease, such as perinatal hypoxia, hydrocephalus and Arnold–Chiari malformation, is present in up to 60% of patients. Diagnosis is established by rigid endoscopy and assessing vocal cord mobility. Management depends upon the severity and progression of the disease. Spontaneous recovery may occur and can take up to 36 months. In the presence of significant airway compromise, tracheostomy will be needed.

Subglottic haemagioma

A **capillary haemangioma** in the subglottis can present between 6 weeks and 6 months of life (Figure 18.8). Cutaneous haemangiomas can be present giving a clue to the diagnosis. Intermittent stridor and a tendency to recurrent episodes of "croup" are noticed. Initially, the haemangioma may grow for a year, after which spontaneous regression occurs. Haemangiomas causing few symptoms can be observed. The mainstay of treatment for infantile haemangiomas is propranolol, a non-selective beta-blocker. The therapeutic effect occurs by vasoconstriction, decreased expression of genes regulating angiogenesis and by triggering apoptosis of capillary endothelial cells. In severe cases, tracheostomy may be needed to maintain the airway until regression, which is usually between 2 and 3 years of

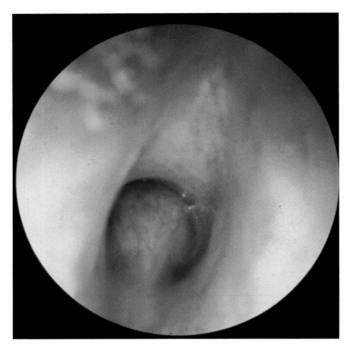

Figure 18.8 Subglottic haemangioma causing airway compromise. (Courtesy of Dr T. McGill, Boston, USA)

age. Other treatment options include laser vaporisation, excision of the haemangioma and systemic steroids may be necessary for partial or non-responders.

Respiratory papillomatosis

This is caused by the human papilloma virus and vertical transmission can occur from the mother to the child during labour. Hoarse voice is the usual presenting symptom, and the airway is compromised in extensive papillomatosis. In the presence of stridor, debulking the papillomatous lesions must be urgently performed to

restore the airway (Figure 18.9). Tracheostomy should be avoided if possible as this can encourage spread of papillomas into the lower airways. Resolution usually occurs towards adolescence. Regular surveillance is needed and debulking or vaporising them with a laser can keep the lesions under control. Addition of topical cidofovir, an antiviral agent, has also been shown to reduce recurrences.

Evaluation of stridor in adults

In the absence of any definite precipitating cause and relevant history, acute and chronic stridor in adults should be considered to be neoplastic unless proven otherwise. A careful history can identify causes such as previous thyroid surgery (bilateral recurrent laryngeal nerve injury, a very rare occurrence these days) and intubation trauma. History of tobacco and alcohol use must be obtained. An assessment of the extent of hypoxia and the work of breathing must be performed as described in Boxes 18.2 and 18.3. It is possible to assess the larynx comprehensively using a flexible nasolaryngoscope and achieve a diagnosis in the outpatient setting in the majority of adults. Based on the extent of decompensation and the diagnosis, observation or intervention must be planned.

Malignancy

Malignant lesions of the larynx and hypopharynx can present with stridor due to direct tumour obstruction of the airway or indirectly by causing vocal cord palsy and oedema (Figure 18.10). It can also occur following radiation to treat laryngeal cancers. It is not possible to secure the airway prior to tracheostomy in all cases, and a local anaesthetic tracheostomy may be needed. Debulking of the tumour to improve the airway while awaiting definitive management is an option in selected cases. The factors that determine treatment are extent of the tumour, coexisting illnesses and patient choice.

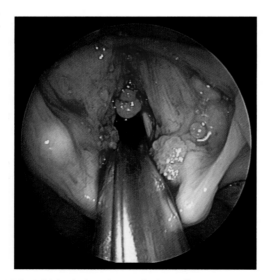

Figure 18.9 Multiple glottis and supraglottic papillomata.

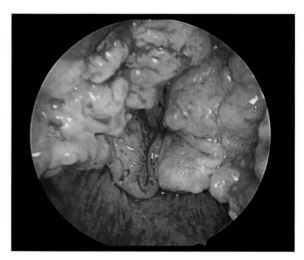

Figure 18.10 Laryngeal cancer causing complete obstruction of the glottis with superficial bleeding caused by intubation.

Definitive treatment options include radiation with or without chemotherapy and surgery. Tumours presenting with stridor are usually well advanced locally and may need total laryngectomy for complete clearance.

Intubation trauma

Intubation for any length of time causes laryngeal inflammation. Extensive inflammation and ulceration can lead to fibrosis and scarring of the airway and can present many weeks later with stridor. This usually occurs in the subglottis. The incidence of these complications is higher with prolonged periods of intubation. Neonates can tolerate intubation for weeks with few long-term effects, but it is reasonable to consider conversion to tracheostomy after 1 week to 10 days of intubation in adults if no extubation is planned. Reconstruction of the stenotic segment is needed in established stenosis to wean the patient off the tracheostomy.

Supraglottitis

Acute supraglottitis in adults behaves differently compared to its course in children. In addition to *H. influenzae*, *Streptococcus pneumoniae* and group A streptococci are also implicated in causation. With a slower onset and odynophagia being the major symptom, airway obstruction is uncommon and it is safe in most instances to perform a flexible endoscopic assessment. Severe sore throat unexplained by significant oropharyngeal findings on examination in adults should prompt a flexible nasolaryngoscopy, which will reveal the diagnosis. Treatment involves inpatient admission with close airway monitoring, antibiotics and intervention as appropriate. There is an increased risk of epiglottic abscess formation and this should be considered if the patient's symptoms do not improve.

Bilateral vocal cord palsy

Although the most common cause of this condition was thyroid surgery in the past, idiopathic causes predominate now. The voice is preserved, with stridor most evident on exertion. Flexible laryngoscopy reveals limitation of abduction of the cords on inspiration. Management options include observation only, a choice of intralaryngeal procedures to increase the airway at the glottic level and tracheostomy. While a tracheostomy preserves the voice very well, all others procedures are designed to increase the glottic airway and avoid a tracheostomy. The voice outcome is likely to be worse with intralaryngeal procedures.

Laryngeal trauma

Blunt and penetrating trauma can cause airway obstruction. Other findings will include hoarseness, subcutaneous emphysema and haemoptysis. In addition to clinical examination, assessment should include cross-sectional imaging. Intubation can cause further disruption to the larynx and the airway is best secured by an urgent tracheostomy. Further treatment to the traumatised larynx is needed as appropriate.

Angioedema

Angioedema is explained by abnormal vascular permeability beneath the dermis. Complement complexes and the kinin system mediate the excessive permeability. The causes of angioedema are set out in Box 18.4. Allergic causes predominate. The onset of oedema can occur within a few hours and in the airway can lead to rapid obstruction. The management is primarily medical with epinephrine, steroids and antihistamines unless caused by C1-esterase inhibitor (C1 INH) deficiency. In the latter, C1 INH concentrates or fresh frozen plasma is required.

Box 18.4 **Causes of angioedema**

- **IgE mediated**: atopy, allergens, physical stimuli
- **Complement mediated**: hereditary (production of low or dysfunctional C1-esterase inhibitor)
- **Non-immunologic**: drug-induced (e.g. angiotensin-converting inhibitors, beta lactam antibiotics)
- **Idiopathic**

Surgical management of the acutely obstructed airway

Whenever possible, children should be transferred to a centre with medical and nursing expertise in managing paediatric airway problems. In children, the airway is secured in conjunction with a direct laryngoscopy. If endotracheal intubation is difficult, a laryngeal mask airway or a rigid bronchoscope can be used to maintain the airway and ventilate the patient while a tracheostomy is performed. A tracheostomy in children, especially neonates, is associated with a high incidence of complications. If rapid deterioration occurs and there is not sufficient time for a tracheostomy, a cricothyrotomy can provide oxygenation until conversion to a tracheostomy. In adults, endotracheal intubation usually is possible in infective and neurologic problems. Adult patients with supraglottitis can usually be observed in a high-dependency setting. Obstructive lesions may need a tracheostomy or debulking of the obstructive lesion.

Tracheostomy

Indications for tracheostomy can be broadly divided into three categories: to bypass the upper airway in airway obstruction; provide pulmonary toilet; and access during head and neck surgery (Figure 18.11). With the exception of severe obstruction seen in neoplastic and traumatic conditions, where the airway cannot be secured from above, this is usually performed under general anaesthesia.

A horizontal incision is made 2 cm above the suprasternal notch. The anterior jugular veins may need to be ligated. Dissection is done in the midline, separating the strap muscles. This will expose the thyroid isthmus, which is ligated and cut. The tracheal rings are exposed and stay sutures are inserted, especially in the

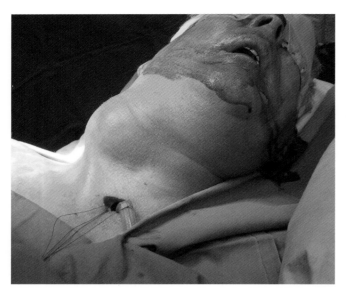

Figure 18.11 Elective tracheostomy performed prior to planned surgical resection of tonsillar squamous cell carcinoma with neck metastases.

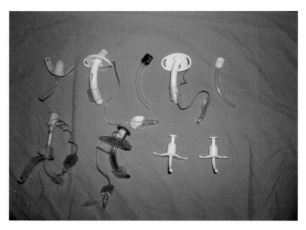

Figure 18.12 Examples of tracheostomy tubes – child and adult, cuffed and uncuffed.

paediatric population. These sutures help with finding the track if the tube were to become displaced in the initial days. A vertical slit tracheostomy is made between the third and fourth rings and the chosen tracheostomy tube inserted. The integrity of the tube and the cuff will need to be checked in advance. The tube is secured in place with sutures and tape as necessary. A tube change is done after 4–7 days, allowing time for the track to mature. An uncuffed tube can be used at this time if there is little concern about significant aspiration.

Tracheostomy tubes

There are several types of tracheostomy tubes available, commonly made of PVC, silicone or silver (Figure 18.12). A cuffed tube is used in the early days after a tracheostomy, especially in the ventilated patient (Figure 18.13). This is usually changed to an uncuffed tube prior to discharge, unless there are significant problems with aspiration. This scenario is commonly seen in patients with neurologic disabilities. A fenestrated tube has a single or multiple holes on the shoulder, allowing phonation when the tube is occluded. Most of the tracheostomy tubes used in hospital and community practice have an inner tube that protrudes just beyond the outer tube at the distal tip. The longer end of the inner tube picks up the dried mucus and can be removed for cleaning, while the outer tube is left in place (Figure 18.13).

Care of the tracheostomy in the community

Patients whose tracheostomy has been performed for chronic airway obstruction or pulmonary toilet may be discharged home with the tracheostomy. Care of the tracheostomy in the community needs significant nursing expertise, as they will be the primary care givers.

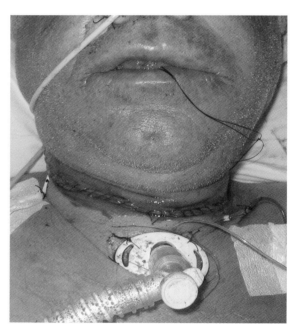

Figure 18.13 Cuffed tracheostomy tube in place to protect airway following surgery of an oropharyngeal cancer.

A good network of communication needs to be in place prior to discharge to ensure that the patient's home is equipped to deal with tracheostomy care. This will include a suction apparatus, a humidification system if required and a supply of spare tracheostomy tubes. The patient's family should be educated regarding tracheostomy care, performing competent suction and replacing the tube in the event of a blockage. Input from a community physiotherapist and speech and language therapist may also be needed. Some problems faced in the community, such as narrowing of the tract and persistent granulations with bleeding around the stoma, may need specialist ENT advice.

Further reading

Bent J. Pediatric laryngotracheal obstruction: current perspectives on stridor. *Laryngoscope* 2006;**116**(7):1059–70.

Peridis S, Pilgrim G, Athanasopoulos I, Parpounas K. A meta-analysis on the effectiveness of propranolol for the treatment of infantile airway haemangiomas. *Int J Pediatr Otorhinolaryngol* 2011;**75**(4):455–60.

Pracy P. Upper airway obstruction, in *Scott-Brown's Otorhinolaryngology, Head and Neck Surgery*, 7th edn, Volume 2, Chapter 174, pp. 2286–304 (ed. M. Gleeson), Hodder Arnold, London, 2008.

Zoumalan R, Maddalozzo J, Holinger LD. Etiology of stridor in infants. *Ann Otol Rhinol Laryngol* 2007;**116**(5):329–34.

CHAPTER 19

Snoring and Obstructive Sleep Apnoea

Tawakir Kamani and Anshul Sama

Nottingham University Hospitals, Queen's Medical Centre Campus, Nottingham, UK

OVERVIEW

- SRBD is a spectrum of conditions ranging from simple snoring to severe OSAHS that develops with increasing reduction in airflow and has a major impact on patient life (socially and medically)

- A major risk factor is obesity and effective strategies to achieve long-term weight loss are desperately needed to curtail the concurrent epidemics of obesity and obstructive sleep apnoea

- The gold standard for diagnosis is polysomnography but this is not always available and other sleep studies are used in conjunction with a detail history (with the patient's partner)and thorough examination

- Treatment of the SRBD depends on its severity and ranges from lifestyle changes and simple surgery amongst simple snorers to mild OSAHS patients whilst patients with moderate to severe OSAHS benefiting from CPAP

- SRBD is common in children and the most common treatment choice for paediatric OSAHS is adenotonsillectomy

---

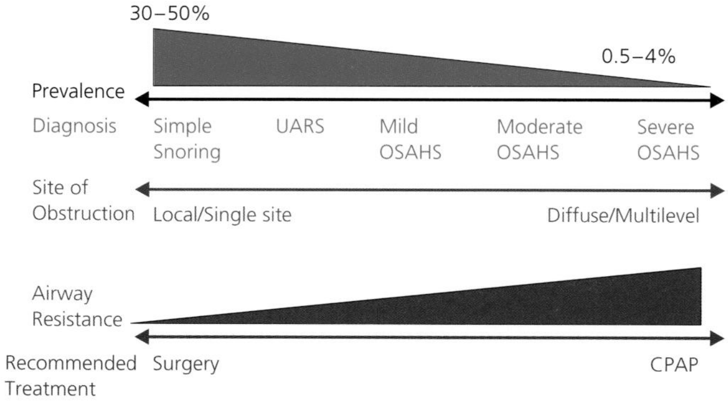

Figure 19.1 The continuum of sleep-disordered breathing. UARS, upper airway resistance syndrome; OSA, obstructive sleep apnoea; OSAHS, obstructive sleep apnoea hypopnea syndrome.

Snoring and obstructive sleep apnoea syndrome (OSAHS) are different degrees of a broadly identified disorder; sleep-related breathing disorder (SRBD). Identifying SRBDs is important as they have a major impact on a patient's life. The medical implications of SRBDs such as increased risk of stroke, hypertension and other cardiovascular conditions such as arrhythmias and myocardial ischaemia are well-documented. Daytime somnolence poses a risk to the individual and public with respect to road traffic accidents. Lastly, marital and relationship disharmony can occur as a consequence of simple snoring; significant improvement in the quality of life is achieved with successful surgery.

Spectrum of the condition

SRBD results from partial or total obstruction of the upper airway. The pathogenesis is multifactorial; reduced muscle tone during sleep and certain anatomical variations in the upper airway predisposing to the condition. Increasing upper airway resistance results in progressive worsening of the disease. SRBD is a spectrum of conditions (Figure 19.1) ranging from simple snoring to severe OSAHS that develops with increasing reduction in airflow.

Depending on the degree of obstruction and associated symptoms, individuals are categorised into one of the following categories:

Simple snoring is categorised by disruptive low frequency sound produced during partial obstruction and vibration of the upper airway without impact on the patient's sleep pattern. This usually arises from soft palate, but the tonsils, epiglottis and the base of the tongue may also contribute in up to 30% of cases. Twenty-five per cent of the population are habitual snorers.

Upper airways resistance syndrome (UARS) is categorised by increased sleep disruption and excessive daytime sleepiness (EDS) without evidence of obstructive apnoeas or de-saturations.

Obstructive sleep apnoea hypopnoea syndrome (OSAHS) is categorised by the coexistence of EDS and interrupted and repeated upper airway collapse during sleep with associated desaturations.

Progression of airway collapse and obstruction leads to either complete with total cessation of airflow (apnoea) or partial with significant hypoventilation (hypopnoea). Severity of OSAHS is determined by frequency of the apnoeas and hypopnoea called the apnoea/hypopnoea index (AHI) (Table 19.1).

Clinically significant OSAHS is only likely to be present when the AHI is greater than 15 events per hour in association with unexplained EDS.

ABC of Ear, Nose and Throat, Sixth Edition.
Edited by Harold Ludman and Patrick J. Bradley.
© 2013 John Wiley & Sons, Ltd. Published 2013 by John Wiley & Sons, Ltd.

Table 19.1 Categories of severity of OSAHS.

Severity of OSAHS	AHI (apnoea/hypopnoea events per hour)
Mild	5–14
Moderate	15–30
Severe	greater than 30

Aetiology

The airway between the posterior end of the nose and the larynx is unprotected by cartilaginous or bony structures and reliant on muscle tone for its patency. SRBD only occurs during sleep when pharyngeal muscle tone falls progressively as sleep condenses to deeper levels. This phenomenon is present in all humans and yet not all humans have SRBD. Abnormalities in both "upper airway" size and muscle activity appear to contribute to its pathogenesis.

Factors found to increase the risk of SRBD are:

Gender – Men have between a twofold and a fivefold increased risk of OSAHS compared with women matched for age and weight. Sex hormones influence upper body obesity and are probably why OSAHS is less common in premenopausal women than postmenopausal women or in men.

Obesity – This is the most important risk factor, and prevalence of SRBD has been shown to directly correlate with the body mass index (BMI). Seventy per cent of individuals with a BMI of 40 or greater suffer with OSAHS. Central obesity indicators such as neck circumference index and waist : hip ratio are recognised as better predictors of OSAHS than BMI.

Obstructive upper airway anatomy – Craniofacial abnormalities are associated with a higher prevalence of SRBD. Features such as retrognathia, tonsillar hypertrophy, enlarged tongue or soft palate, inferiorly positioned hyoid bone, maxillary and mandibular retroposition, and decreased posterior airway space can narrow upper airway dimensions and promote the occurrence of OSAHS during sleep. Decreased nasal airway due to turbinate hypertrophy, septal deviations or nasal polyposis increases upper airway resistance and can contribute, but is unlikely to be the sole cause for SRBD.

Other risk factors – given in Table 19.2.

Consequences of sleep-related breathing disorders

Simple snoring has a significant social impact but no detrimental impact on the individual's health. Conversely, OSAHS results in significant cardiovascular and neurocognitive consequences.

Neurocognitive effects – Sleep fragmentation results in EDS (commonest complaint) in patients with OSAHS. Cognitive performance is notably impaired with deterioration in memory, intellectual capacity and motor co-ordination. Patients with OSAHS have a significant increase in accident rates with 20% of road traffic accidents on major highways caused by sleepiness at the wheel.

Cardiovascular consequences – OSAHS is associated and contributes to systemic hypertension. Treatment with continuous positive

Table 19.2 Other associated risk factors of OSAHS.

Risk factor	Associations	Salient points
Age	Progressive increase in prevalence of SRBD in 6-7th decades	Narrower and possibly more collapsible upper airways seen with increasing age
Hereditary	Two- to fourfold greater	In first degree relatives
Medical history	Hypothyroidism Acromegaly Neuromuscular diseases Chronic lung disease* (*not a direct risk for SRBD)	Due to craniofacial anomaly Central apnoeas are more likely OSAHS is more severe with deeper events de-saturation due to hypo-ventilation and lower lung reserve
Social history	Smoking Alcohol	
Drugs	Hypnotics Opioids	Central depression increase the risk of SRBD

airway pressure (CPAP) reduces blood pressure (BP) which decreases cardiac events by 20% and stroke risk by 40% over 5–10 years. OSAHS is also associated with cerebrovascular disease.

Metabolic syndrome – OSAHS is associated with major metabolic impairment caused by higher blood pressure, and poorer lipid and glucose control, independent of central obesity or type 2 diabetes mellitus.

Others – An increased likelihood of impotence and gastro-oeosophageal reflux have been known in patients with OSAHS.

Assessment

Clinical assessment of SRBD entails a detailed history, ideally with the partner present during the consultation. The aims of the history, clinical examination and investigations are given as follows.

Identify if the patient has OSAHS

All suspected OSAHS patients and their partners should complete an Epworth sleepiness scale (ESS) to subjectively assess the degree of sleepiness. ESS is a validated method of identifying EDS. Although the correlation between ESS and OSAHS severity is relatively weak, the ESS is used as a guide for the clinician to the patient's perception of his/her sleepiness.

Identify predisposing factors

A through physical examination of nasal airway and pharyngeal anatomy (oropharyngeal inlet including tonsil, tongue and mandibular size) is essential preferably with an endoscope. However, there is poor correlation between clinical findings and predictability of OSAHS. A medical history to identify risk factors such as hypothyroidism should always be obtained.

Formal sleep studies confirm the clinical suspicion and severity of OSAHS in order to guide the therapeutic choices to offer patients. OSAHS is present in over 30% of snorers without symptoms of EDS and should always be excluded in all patients before considering

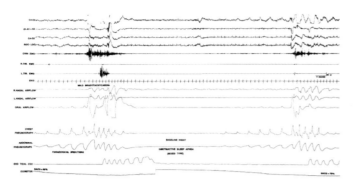

Figure 19.2 Polysomnography trace.

surgery for snoring as uvulopalatopharyngoplasty (UPPP) may compromise future CPAP therapy. Patients with COPD and snoring should have an urgent sleep study as its combination with severe OSAHS is potentially dangerous. All patients who drive long distances, heavy goods vehicles or handle hazardous machinery as part of their profession must have a sleep study as part of their assessment.

Investigation of snoring and sleep apnoea involves the use of one or all of the following different sleep studies:

Polysomnography (PSG) – The gold standard for diagnosis of OSAHS. This entails an inpatient study involving overnight assessment of variable number of parameters including-EEG, electromyogram, electro-oculogram, respiratory airflow, thoracoabdominal movement, ECG, oximetry, body position, snoring sound and video. It is a relatively intrusive and costly study whose interpretation can be complex (Figure 19.2).

Ambulatory pulse oximetry – This is useful for OSAHS screening. It has good specificity and positive predictive value but poor sensitivity and negative predictive value. Therefore, it is useful only in the presence of a positive result oximetry.

Limited sleep studies – These usually incorporate some measurement of respiratory signals such as airflow, thoracoabdominal movement, oximetry and pulse measurement. These studies can be performed at home and are common practice in the UK. Disadvantages include inability to identify sleep stages, conditions such as restless leg syndrome, equipment failure and night to night repeatability. Whilst these concerns are appreciated, limited studies can be useful, cost effective and an accepted method of assessment.

Localise the level(s) of obstruction in the upper airway

Radiological imaging – Studying upper airway size or shape by computed tomography, magnetic resonance imaging, or cephalometry does not accurately differentiate patients with OSAHS from normal subjects and cannot be recommended in the routine assessment of patients with possible OSAHS. These are useful if mandibular or maxillary surgery is planned.

Pharyngeal manometry – This involves pressure transducers within catheters placed in the pharynx and oesophagus to determine pressure measurements at different levels within the upper airway and proven superior in identification of site of obstruction and

can be performed concurrent with sleep studies. There is limited evidence that manometry data can be used in isolation to identify successful surgical candidates.

Sleep (sedation) nasendoscopy – Different levels of the upper airway are visualised simultaneously. Sedation is used to induce pharyngeal muscle tone relaxation to simulate sleep with a patient in supine position. Once sedated, a nasendoscope is passed and events of obstruction and patterns of vibration observed. The information they give is limited as these are not performed during natural sleep and unipositional. Its main use is to evaluate the appropriateness of oropharyngeal surgery.

Treatment options

The choice of treatment is dictated by:

- diagnosis (Table 19.3)
- accurate localisation of the level of airway obstruction.

The efficacy of the treatment is dependent on accurate localisation of the site of obstruction. Fibre optic upper airway endoscopy, with our without sedation and pharyngeal manometry are helpful but have limitations as in the information that they provide as discussed above.

Conservative treatment measures

Behavioural changes – This includes simple measures such as allowing the partner to fall asleep first, using ear plugs, or sleeping on your side rather than the back can often suffice.

Weight loss – This has been shown to improve SRBD symptoms. The most dramatic results have been reported with surgical weight loss. It should be recognised, that substantial weight loss by non surgical means is both difficult to achieve and hard to maintain.

Lifestyle changes – While smoking is linked with OSAHS, there is no evidence that stopping smoking improves apnoeic events. Alcohol exaggerates loss of pharyngeal muscle tone during sleep and episodes of airway collapse. Similarly, sleeping tablets, sedative antihistamines and tranquillizers should be avoided at bedtime.

Table 19.3 Treatment options dependant on diagnostic degree of SRBD.

Diagnosis spectrum of SRBD	Aim of treatment	Treatment options
Simple snoring	Reduce snoring to socially acceptable levels	Life style changes, weight loss, oral devices and limited surgery
UARS and mild OSAHS	Reduce snoring, upper airway resistance and associated sleep fragmentation	Depends on patient choice and predominant symptom – snoring noise or sleep disturbance
Moderate to severe OSAHS	Eliminating episodes of apnoeas/hypopnoea, de-saturations, and EDS.	Gold standard treatment is use of CPAP

Intraoral appliance – Several types are available. These increase pharyngeal airway by moving and fixing the mandible forward. These devices are effective in improving snoring and mild OSAHS. A significant proportion (60–65%) of patients report side effects such as excessive salivation, jaw discomfort, teeth/gum discomfort and temporomandibular joint dysfunction.

CPAP – This is the most effective treatment for OSAHS. It eliminates apnoea/hypopnoea, improves daytime alertness, neurocognitive functions, mood and cardiovascular sequelae. CPAP suffers from notable compliance limitations. Approximately, one third of patients offered CPAP are unwilling to use it and average nocturnal use averages between 4–5 hours per night. Compliance can be improved by initial habituation to the mask for several days before CPAP usage, eliminating oral leakage with chin straps, using nasal cushions to reduce claustrophobia, heated humidification to reduce nasal dryness, bi-level positive airway pressure or Auto-CPAP to reduce exhalation pressure. Often the most important factor is supportive and accessible medical staff.

Pharmacological treatments

These include respiratory stimulants that increase upper airway muscle tone, or drugs for treating excessive daytime hypersomnolence. Protrytyline, acetozalaminde and progesterone are respiratory stimulants and also suppress rapid eye movement sleep (the sleep stage most prone to airway collapse), but are not curative in the treatment of OSAHS. Addition of alerting drugs such as modafanil, may have some effect on reducing daytime sleepiness in patients who remain sleepy despite CPAP usage. Its use cannot be considered as an alternative to CPAP as it fails to address the underlying pathology of OSAHS and associated complications.

Upper airway surgery

Successful surgery depends on accurate identification of the level(s) of obstruction and on choice of surgical treatment effective for addressing that level(s) of obstruction. Current surgical approaches are designed to widen the upper airway – nasal, oropharyngeal or retrolingual. These procedures are usually single site and non-invasive for simple snoring or multiple level and invasive for moderate to severe OSAHS.

Tracheostomy was the first surgical procedure used in the treatment of OSAHS. Although completely effective, it is rarely performed due to associated morbidities.

Nasal surgery to address deviated septum, nasal polyposis and turbinate hypertrophy can significantly reduce upper airway resistance. However, the reported impact on snoring is variable with a known relapse after several years. Depending upon the severity of OSAHS, nasal airway reconstruction may contribute to decreased CPAP level and improvement in oxygen saturation and should be considered in the overall management of OSAHS.

Uvulopalatopharyngoplasty involves tonsillectomy, uvulectomy and excision of a variable segment of the soft palate (Figure 19.3). Success rates for simple snoring vary between 75 and 85%

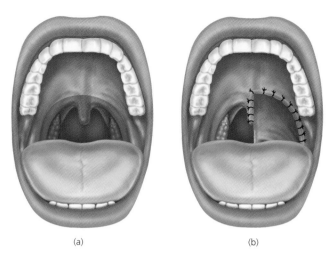

(a)   (b)

Figure 19.3 Traditional UPPP: (a) surgical outline of UPPP; (b) left side UPPP complete.

and for OSAHS are 52.3%, with success rate decreasing with time.

Laser-assisted uvulopalatoplasty (LAUP) developed as a modification of the traditional UPPP. Its reported success rate is between 51–89% dependent on the time of follow up. Studies show that LAUP is more effective than doing nothing in OSAHS but less effective than conventional UPPP.

Radiofrequency (RF) procedures of the tonsil, palate and tongue base involve submucosal application of low frequency radiowaves to create thermic lesions and subsequent volume reduction and scarring. Its advantages include mucosal sparing and emphasis on volume reduction and scarring rather than resection. Approximate 80% reduction in subjective snoring at 1 year with prolonged improvement in daytime somnolence, OSAS-related quality of life, psychomotor vigilance, and AHI is achieved.

Maxillofacial and multilevel surgery performed for patients with moderate to severe OSAHS includes a range of procedures to improve the retrolingual airway and the retropalatal airway. Although invasive, this is the most effective treatment for OSAHS after tracheostomy with comparable reduction of AHI compared to CPAP, with 90% success after 51 months.

Snoring and obstructive sleep apnoea in children

SRBD is common in children; 3–12% of children snore, while OSAHS affects 1–10% of children that snore. The incidence is equal in both sexes and does not increase with age. The peak occurrence is between the ages of 2 and 5 years, when the adenoids and tonsils are largest in relation to the oropharyngeal size.

Snoring is the commonest symptom in children under 5 years. Other symptoms are summarised in Box 19.1. Paradoxically, children often demonstrate restlessness and hyperactivity, whilst sleepiness is less of a problem compared to adults. Resolution of these symptoms after successful treatment suggests causation. Medical sequelae such as systemic hypertension, cor pulomonale and congestive heart failure are rare and associated with severe cases.

Box 19.1 **Other common symptoms of OSAHS in children**

- Mouth breathing
- Diaphoresis
- Restlessness
- Frequent awakenings
- Witnessed apnoeic episodes
- Enuresis
- Behaviour problems
- Deficient attention span
- Failure to thrive
- Restlessness and hyperactivity

Pathophysiology

Most children with OSAHS will present with adenotonsillar hypertrophy with narrowed oropharyngeal airway. However, many children with documented adenotonsillar hypertrophy never have symptoms of OSAHS suggesting a complex interplay between adenotonsillar hypertrophy and loss of neuromuscular tone.

Children with craniofacial syndromes such as choanal stenosis/atresia, macroglossia, micrognathia, mid face hypoplasia (e.g. Down syndrome, Crouzon's syndrome) and mandibular hypoplasia (e.g. Pierre Robin syndrome) have fixed anatomic variations predisposing them to airway obstruction, while hypotonia causes obstruction in children with neuromuscular disease.

Investigation and treatment

The use of polysomnography in children in the UK is infrequent. An AHI of >1 is considered abnormal. History and examination are good predictors of childhood SRBD. Overnight oximetry is the commonest screening tool and recommended in all children before considering surgery. Adenotonsillectomy remains the treatment of choice for most children and is noted to resolve clinical symptoms in up to 73% of children with AHI of more than 10 before surgery.

CPAP is indicated when adenotonsillectomy is contraindicated or failed; 20% of children find CPAP difficult to tolerate. Surgical management of craniofacial syndromes and OSAHS requires more than standard adenotonsillectomy, and tracheostomy is often necessary.

The natural course and long-term prognosis of childhood OSAHS are unknown. It is not known whether childhood OSAHS is a precursor of adult OSAHS or two diverse diseases affecting discrete populations.

Further reading

Chan J, Edman J, Koltai PJ. Obstructive sleep apnea in children. *Am Fam Physician* 2004;**69**:1147–54.

Lim J, McKean M. Adenotonsillectomy for obstructive sleep apnea in children. *Cochrane Database Syst Rev* 2003;Issue 4:CD003136.

Management of Obstructive Sleep Apnoea/Hypopnoea Syndrome in Adults. A National Clinical Guideline. Scottish Intercollegiate Guideline network, June 2003, www.sign.ac.uk

Ulualp SO. Snoring and obstructive sleep apnea. *Med Clin Nth Am* 2010; **94**(5): 1047–55.

Young T, Peppard PE, Gottlieb OJ. Epidemiology of obstructive sleep apnea: a population health perspective. *Am J Resp Critical Care Med* 2002; **165**: 1217–39.

CHAPTER 20

Swallowing Problems

Vinidh Paleri[1] and Patrick J. Bradley[2]

[1]Newcastle upon Tyne Hospitals, Newcastle, UK
[2]Nottingham University Hospitals, Queen's Medical Centre Campus, Nottingham, UK

> ## OVERVIEW
>
> - Dysphagia is the symptom of swallowing impairment
> - There are four stages of swallowing: oral preparatory, oral, pharyngeal and oesophageal
> - Weight loss, when associated with dysphagia, indicates significant disease and needs urgent investigation
> - Aspiration is defined as liquids or solids penetrating below the level of the vocal cords, and can be associated with both neurologic and neoplastic conditions
> - Multidisciplinary evaluation may be necessary for diagnosis, treatment and rehabilitation

Dysphagia is a symptom experienced when there is an impairment or alteration of the swallowing mechanism leading to difficulty moving food and liquid through the mouth, pharynx or oesophagus. This should be differentiated from globus pharyngeus, where there is a sensation of irritation, tightness or foreign body in the throat, usually noticed at rest and is not affected or relieved by pharyngeal movement. Dysphagia can be an indicator of disease in body systems, from neurological through to hormonal and metabolic. Department of Health figures for 2010–11 record more than 34 000 primary diagnoses of dysphagia in the UK.

Physiology

The swallowing action can be divided into four stages: oral preparatory, oral, pharyngeal and oesophageal. The **oral preparatory stage** is under voluntary control and good motor control of the facial and lingual musculature is essential. It is characterised by increased tone of the lip, buccal and facial muscles, lateral jaw motion and rolling movement of the tongue from side to side that moves the food bolus for mastication. The **oral stage** is also under voluntary control, when the tongue pushes the prepared food bolus towards the oropharynx. Contact of the bolus with the anterior tonsillar pillar is traditionally thought of as the trigger point to initiate the pharyngeal stage. The oral stage lasts approximately between 1 and 1.5 s. Tongue movement plays the most important part in these two stages.

The **pharyngeal stage** (Figure 20.1) lasts only a second, but is accompanied by numerous neuromuscular activities controlled at the brainstem level. The soft palate closes against the nasopharynx to prevent nasal regurgitation and laryngeal closure occurs to prevent aspiration. Three tiers are involved in laryngeal closure, including the epiglottis and the aryepiglottic folds, the false cords and the true cords. Adduction of the true cords occurs before the other tiers (although there may be individual variation) and plays an important role in airway protection. The epiglottis may play a greater role in directing the bolus into the piriform sinuses than in protecting the airway. Surgical resection of the upper two tiers alone is compatible with aspiration-free swallowing as they can learn to compensate by using an airway protection technique (see therapy). Following laryngeal closure, the pharyngeal constrictor muscles sequentially begin contracting to propel the bolus. The

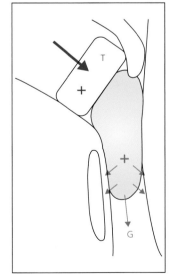 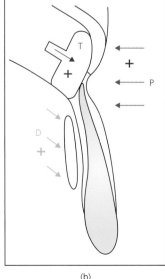

(a)   (b)

Figure 20.1 Pharyngeal phase of swallowing: (a) early phase. (b) late phase. D, depression; E, elevation; G, gravity; T, tongue; +, positive pressure; −, negative pressure.

ABC of Ear, Nose and Throat, Sixth Edition.
Edited by Harold Ludman and Patrick J. Bradley.
© 2013 John Wiley & Sons, Ltd. Published 2013 by John Wiley & Sons, Ltd.

suprahyoid muscles elevate the larynx, clearing the bolus down and the cricopharyngeal sphincter opens, admitting the bolus into the upper oesophagus. The resting tone of the cricopharyngeus reduces with laryngeal elevation and upward movement of the larynx mechanically pulls opens the sphincter and is further opened by bolus pressure. The **oesophageal stage** is of variable duration, lasting between 8 and 20 s.

Symptoms

Swallowing problems can present as difficulty in initiating the swallow, choking or coughing upon swallowing (aspiration), or a sensation of obstruction at the level of the neck or behind the sternum. Dysphagia can be a problem with solids or liquids or both. Dysphagia that is limited to solids initially, progresses to liquids over a period of weeks to months, and is accompanied by weight loss raises suspicion of a malignant lesion. Very slow progression over years occurs in achalasia of the cardia and pharyngeal pouches (Zenker's diverticula), associated with regurgitation of undigested food. Dry mouth (xerostomia) caused by autoimmune diseases (e.g. Sjögren's syndrome) and radiation therapy also causes dysphagia.

Weakness of the oral and lingual musculature can lead to drooling and poor mastication. Altered sensation to the pharynx caused centrally (e.g. neurologic disease) or peripherally (e.g. postradiotherapy), can lead to a delay in the initiation of the pharyngeal stage, and food can slip into the oropharynx. This can cause aspiration, as the airway is unprotected except for a very short time during the pharyngeal stage. Aspiration usually manifests as coughing and choking episodes, or a 'wet' voice quality. Aspiration can also be caused if any of the laryngeal protective mechanisms are impaired, commonly due to neurologic or neoplastic processes. The severity of the problem will dictate the symptomatology. Minor aspiration is characterised by throat clearing and coughing after swallowing, while significant aspiration can cause choking episodes and pneumonitis. Silent aspiration can also occur in the absence of any of the above symptoms, when laryngeal sensation is impaired.

Clinical evaluation

The aim of clinical examination is to assess the swallowing performance and establish the cause of dysphagia. A careful history is required regarding onset of the problem, the severity of dysphagia, weight loss, aspiration, regurgitation and dysphonia. The history can give good pointers towards the diagnosis in 80% to 85% of patients. Acute dysphagia is usually caused by foreign bodies. Meat boluses may pass spontaneously, but most others will need endoscopic management. Dysphagia of longer than three weeks duration needs specialist referral (Figure 20.2). A comprehensive otolaryngologic examination is mandatory, and this includes a flexible fibreoptic assessment of the nasopharynx, hypopharynx and larynx. Lesions in the apex of the pyriform sinus and the postcricoid region may not be evident on flexible endoscopy.

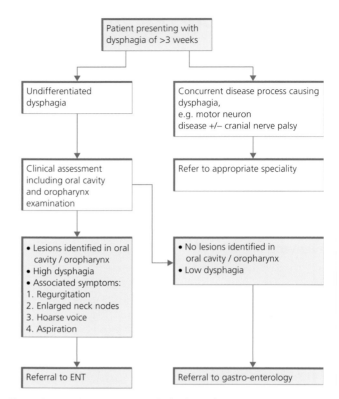

Figure 20.2 Patient presenting with dysphagia for > 3 weeks.

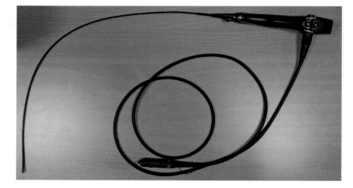

Figure 20.3 Transnasal flexible oesophagoscope.

Transnasal flexible oesophagoscopy (TNO) (Figure 20.3) is being increasingly used by otolaryngologists to evaluate dysphagia. This offers a one-stop service to evaluate the postcricoid region and the oesophagus, obviating routine use of rigid endoscopy under general anaesthesia in many patients. The presence of significant findings in the oesophagus can be followed up by referral to gastroenterology. Contrast swallows are useful in identifying the presence and size of pharyngeal pouches and oesophageal dysmotility. Videofluoroscopy is a multidisciplinary, dynamic assessment of the anatomy and co-ordination of the oral, pharyngeal and oesophageal stages of swallowing. The flow chart in Figure 20.4 shows an algorithmic approach to referral from primary care and also identifies the role of various investigations in the diagnosis of dysphagia.

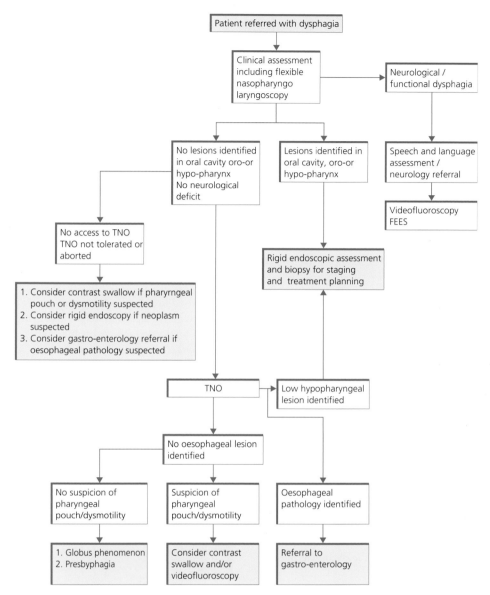

Figure 20.4 Patient referred with dysphagia (ENT assessment).

Common otolaryngologic conditions causing chronic dysphagia

The various conditions encountered in routine clinical practice are shown in Figure 20.5 and some discussed below in detail.

Presbyphagia

Physiologic changes occur in the swallowing reflex with ageing, and accompanied by reduction in muscle mass and strength, can cause dysphagia. Presentation is that of a chronic dysphagia with malnutrition and aspiration. Clinical examination is often unhelpful and investigation is needed to exclude other causes of dysphagia common in this population. Treatment involves modifying the consistency of food and swallowing therapy along with correction of other concurrent contributory factors.

Globus pharyngeus

Globus pharyngeus is a sensation of lump or tightness in the throat, where no organic cause is identified. Aetiologic hypotheses for globus include atypical manifestation of gastro-oesophageal reflux, oesophageal dysmotility and psychogenic origin. The presentation is usually in middle age and although the sensation is equally prevalent in both sexes, women seek medical attention more often. Diagnosis is based on the clinical history and findings: lack of true dysphagia, no weight loss, intermittent symptoms typically maximum between meals and a continual need to swallow. Examination should include

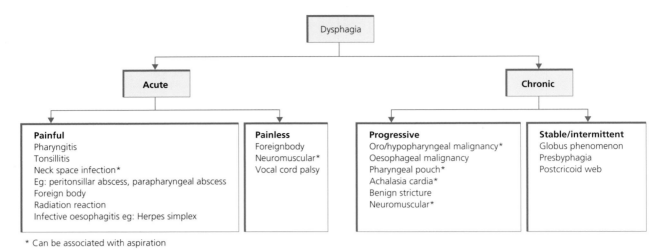

* Can be associated with aspiration

Figure 20.5 Flow chart showing the differential diagnostic options for dysphagia of otolaryngological origin.

a flexible nasolaryngoscopy and transnasal oesophagoscopy, and this is typically normal. Unless the presentation is atypical, further investigation is unwarranted. Treatment involves reassurance and an explanation of the problem, with antireflux therapy if reflux is present. These symptoms can last for at least 2 years with 45% experiencing symptoms for up to 7 years.

Pharyngeal pouch (Zenker's diverticulum):

An area of natural weakness occurs in the posterior aspect of the hypopharynx, between the fibres of the thyropharyngeus and the cricopharyngeus muscles (upper oesophageal sphincter) of the inferior pharyngeal constrictor. Pulsion diverticula can form at this site, where the divergence of the fibres lends less support to the pharyngeal wall (Figure 20.6). There is no consensus on the aetiology of pharyngeal pouches, but various hypotheses include poor relaxation of the cricopharyngeal muscle during swallowing, increased resting tone of the muscle and myopathy of the cricopharyngeus.

This condition is usually seen in the elderly and presents with progressive dysphagia and weight loss. Symptoms include regurgitation of undigested food many hours after eating, gurgling sounds in the neck during swallowing, halitosis and coughing episodes with aspiration. Endoscopic examination may reveal some pooling of residue in the hypopharynx and reflux, called the "rising tide" sign. A contrast swallow establishes diagnosis (Figure 20.7). These patients are prone to oesophageal perforation during endoscopic examination if the pouch is not recognised pre-operatively. Treatment depends on the size of the pouch and the symptoms. Small pouches discovered incidentally can be observed. The management of choice for larger, symptomatic pouches is endoscopic stapling

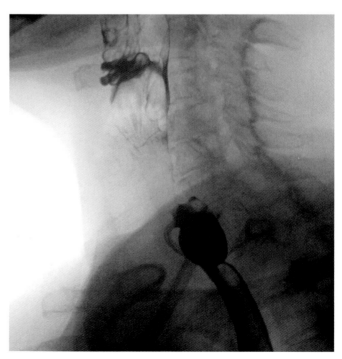

Figure 20.7 Radiological image of a "large pharyngeal pouch".

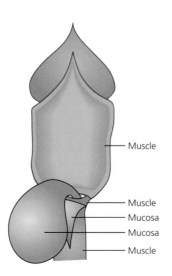

Figure 20.6 Anatomy of a pharyngeal pouch.

Figure 20.8 How a pharyngeal pouch is stapled (endoscopic cricopharyngeal myotomy): (a) a prominent cricopharyngeal "bar" muscle, the oesophageal opening anteriorly and the pouch posteriorly; (b) the method of stapling, with two rows of three sets of staples, between which the muscle and the mucosa are divided; (c) the bar has been divided – increasing the opening into the oesophagus.

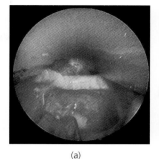
(a)

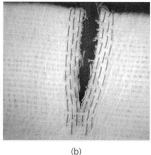
(b)

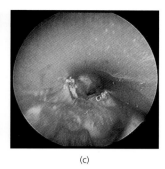
(c)

of the party wall between the pouch and the oesophagus to prevent food from stagnating in the pouch (Figure 20.8). There is a very small incidence of malignancy in these pouches and careful telescopic inspection is essential prior to stapling. Difficult exposure due to short neck and anteriorly placed larynx may preclude stapling, when an external approach is required to excise the pouch.

Postcricoid web

This condition is usually seen in women in the fourth and fifth decades of life, in association with iron deficiency anaemia and weight loss, although the incidence is decreasing. The onset is gradual and patients have altered dietary habits at presentation to compensate for the dysphagia. Examination findings may include cheilitis and atrophic tongue (Figure 20.9) from iron deficiency. Diagnosis is established by the finding of a perpendicular, thin filling defect, usually arising on the anterior wall. While early webs may be reversible with iron supplementation, the majority need rigid endoscopic dilatation of the web for symptomatic relief. The significance of these webs is unclear. Postcricoid carcinoma, unlike at other hypopharyngeal subsites, is more common in younger women and one-third to two-thirds of these patients have experienced symptoms of a web.

Malignancy of the oropharynx and hypopharynx

The tonsils, base of tongue, soft palate and the posterior pharyngeal wall down to the level of the hyoid bone comprise the regions of the oropharynx. The hypopharynx starts at the level of the hyoid and extends to the inferior border of the cricoid cartilage and includes the following subsites: the piriform fossae, posterior pharyngeal wall and postcricoid region (Figure 20.10)

Squamous cell carcinomas are the most common neoplastic lesions in this region. Verrucous carcinomas, malignancies arising from the minor salivary glands and lymphomas are also seen. The following discussion will focus only on squamous cancer, as it accounts for more than 90% of malignancies in this region.

Dysphagia associated with malignant tumours is progressive and likely to be associated with weight loss. Late presentation is the norm, especially for hypopharyngeal carcinomas, as small lesions tend to be asymptomatic. Other head and neck symptoms are often present including dysphonia caused by vocal cord palsy and/or aspiration, referred otalgia, neck metastases and airway compromise. Clinical examination is helpful in identifying the primary site, but rigid endoscopy under general anaesthesia is needed to carefully map out the extent of the tumour. CT or MRI of the neck and chest helps to stage the disease and plan management.

Single modality treatment, surgery or radiation therapy usually suffices for early lesions. Early and selected advanced tumours of the oropharynx and hypopharynx can be removed transorally under microscopic control using the laser (Figures 20.11 and 20.12). This technique reduces morbidity in contrast to the conventional open approach. Swallowing difficulties after treatment for small tumours may be short-lived. Advanced oropharyngeal tumours are usually treated by organ preservation approaches with salvage surgery as appropriate. Advanced staged hypopharyngeal tumours, especially with laryngeal invasion and significant dysphagia are

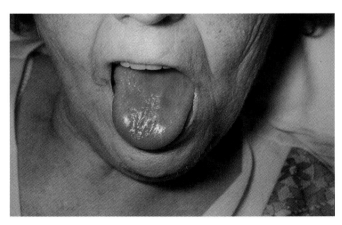

Figure 20.9 Angular chelitis and atrophic stomatitis.

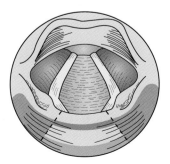

Figure 20.10 Regions of the hypopharynx (purple, piriform sinus; blue, postcricoid space; green, posterior pharyngeal wall).

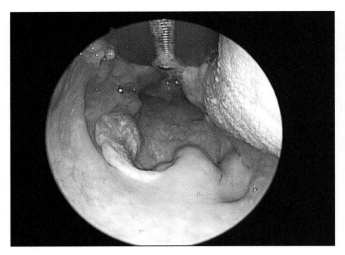

Figure 20.11 Early left tonsil (oropharyngeal) cancer.

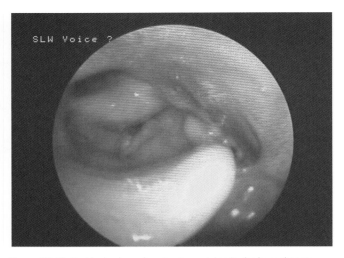

Figure 20.13 Residual coloured contrast remaining in the hypopharynx.

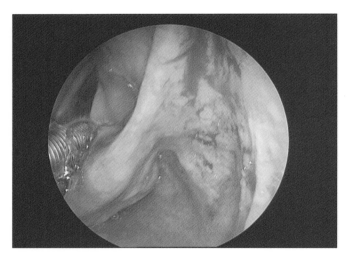

Figure 20.12 Small tumour located anterolateral of the right piriform fossa (hypopharynx).

more likely to benefit from a primary surgical approach. Significant nursing, nutritional and swallowing support is necessary for patients receiving concurrent chemoradiation.

Neurologic diseases

Myasthenia gravis, multiple sclerosis, motor neurone disease, muscular dystrophies and other degenerative disorders can affect swallowing. The problem occurs with initiation of the swallow for both solids and liquids, and these symptoms are usually progressive. Based on the severity of the underlying problem swallowing therapy may be helpful. These patients are also prone to aspiration due to diminished sensation to the pharynx and impaired lingual muscle and pharyngeal constrictor activity. Where aspiration is

intractable and the patient is having difficulty maintaining their daily calorific intake, alternative or augmentative tube feeding (i.e. surgically placed gastrostomy) may be considered.

Acute onset palsy of the vagus can present with dysphagia, aspiration (Figure 20.13) and a breathy voice. The aetiology is often idiopathic, with possible causes being viral neuritis and damage to the neural microvasculature by underlying systemic causes such as diabetes mellitus. Structural lesions must be ruled out by imaging the course of the recurrent laryngeal nerve from the skull base to the diaphragm for left cord palsy and to the superior mediastinum for right cord palsy. Improvement in symptoms may take place by compensation provided by the contralateral cord over a few months. A head turn to the affected side on swallowing can be effective in reducing aspiration. If aspiration continues with poor speech, the affected cord can be medialised surgically to meet the other cord, thus reducing aspiration and improving the voice.

Percutaneous gastrostomy (PG)

High-dose radiation therapy to the primary site and neck in the setting of cancer-related dysphagia, especially when combined with concurrent chemotherapy, can lead to severe mucositis and restriction in oral intake. Supplementation of feeds by nasogastric tube or PG is needed. The PG is inserted prior to starting treatment under endoscopic, ultrasound or fluoroscopic guidance without the need for a laparotomy (Figure 20.14). It is easily performed with minimal morbidity. Complications include wound infection and rarely metastasis (less than 1%) at the gastrostomy site, the latter seen only with the endoscopic technique. It is advantageous in giving the patient more mobility, as the wide lumen enables faster feeding times, and better cosmesis and comfort compared to nasogastric tubes. PG is also widely used in neurologic practice, where long-term dysphagia is expected.

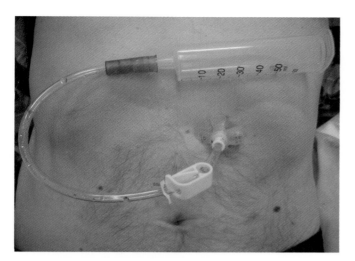

Figure 20.14 Percutaneous gastrostomy.

Swallowing therapy

Speech and Language Therapists (SaLT) may be involved in the diagnosis, rehabilitation and ongoing monitoring and support of patients with oro-pharyngeal dysphagia. Following clinical assessment and videofluroscopy or endosocopic assessment when indicated, the SaLT may recommend a number of management or rehabilitation strategies aimed at improving nutritional status, prevention of chest infections or pneumonia, and maximising quality of life. Common interventions may include head or body postures helping to improve the control and direction of bolus flow, manoeuvres such as those designed to improve airway closure and protection or the efficiency of bolus clearance, exercises to increase the range or strength of movements of the swallowing musculature and/or dietary modifications to suit the patient's abilities. Recommendations may also be made regarding the need for alternative or supplementary nutrition and excluding or reducing oral intake; psychological support may also be provided.

Further reading

Amin MR, Postma GN, Setzen M, Koufman JA. Transnasal esophagoscopy: a position statement from the American Bronchoesophagological Association (ABEA). *Otolaryngol Head Neck Surg* 2008;**138**(4):411–4.

Leslie P, Carding PN, Wilson JA. Investigation and management of chronic dysphagia. *BMJ* 2003;**326**:433–6.

Spieker MR. Evaluating dysphagia. *Am Fam Physician* 2000;**61**:3639–48.

CHAPTER 21

Head and Neck Trauma

Paul Tierney

Southmead Hospital, Westbury-on-Trym, Bristol, UK

OVERVIEW

- Traumatic injury to nasal or septum causing haematoma should be drained to prevent cartilage destruction and subsequent deformity

- Nasal fractures can be manipulated back into position within 3 weeks of an injury. A delay of treatment beyond this time will allow the fracture to heal and any correction of deformity will require a rhinoplasty

- Traumatic perforations of the tympanic membrane should be managed conservatively, but all cases of middle or inner ear injury should undergo audiological and neurological assessment

- An injury to the facial area, blunt or penetrating, that results in a facial nerve weakness requires urgent specialist evaluation

- Major trauma to the head and neck requires stabilisation of airway and cervical spine as a priority

- Vascular injuries in the head and neck may be occult and a high index of suspicion will guide investigation

- Aphonia after neck injury may indicate severe laryngeal injury and impending loss of airway

A patient presenting with trauma to the head and neck region should undergo a thorough and complete examination with assessment and stabilisation of airway, breathing and circulation as a first priority.

The most common injuries to the head and neck involve blunt trauma. Motor vehicle accidents, assaults and sporting injuries commonly cause blunt trauma. However lacerations to soft tissues and penetrating injuries may also occur. A penetrating injury may initially seem trivial but the trauma could be significant with injury to the brain, orbital contents, facial nerve, aerodigestive tract, neurological or vascular structures.

Nasal injury

Nasal injury is commonly due to blunt trauma. A deviation of the nasal bones and septum can give rise to symptoms of nasal blockage

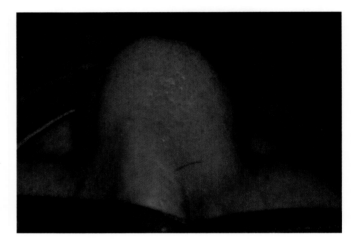

Figure 21.1 Nasal deformity.

and give rise to a significant cosmetic deformity (Figure 21.1). An injury to the cartilaginous and bony septum should be assessed to exclude a septal haematoma. This injury is more common in children as the mucoperichondrium is less well bound to the cartilage. If left untreated, the haematoma may become infected leading to abscess formation or a septal perforation.

An initial evaluation of the extent of a nasal injury may not be possible due to swelling. The patient is commonly seen 5 days after injury, so a full functional and cosmetic assessment may take place. A deviated and impacted nasal bone may be elevated back into position provided the manipulation is performed within 14–21 days after injury. If treatment is delayed beyond this time, fixation of the bones will occur and corrective surgery by nasal osteotomies will be needed in the form of a rhinoplasty. Uncomplicated septal deviations may be treated by a septoplasty operation.

Any patient presenting with a nasal injury should be assessed for the possibility of a facial fracture. Oedema may make examination difficult but palpation of the orbital rims and zygomatic arches should be undertaken with note taken of any tenderness, irregularities or steps. The eyes should be examined to exclude any evidence of injury to the globe, optic nerve or ocular movement. Fractures involving the orbital floor can trap orbital fat or extra ocular muscles, a classical blow-out fracture (Figure 21.2). If fat

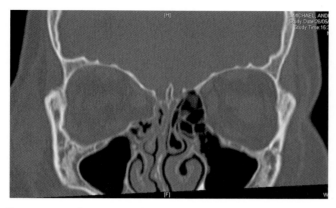

Figure 21.2 CT illustrating a right orbital fracture or a "blow-out" fracture.

is trapped then enopthalmus may be noted but entrapment of muscles can lead to diplopia.

Plain X-rays are rarely needed for the assessment of nasal fractures. However, radiological assessment of facial injury should involve CT scanning if there is any suspicion of a fracture involving the zygoma or orbital floor.

Ear trauma

All patients who are suspected of sustaining a significant trauma to the middle or inner ear or temporal bone should have a hearing assessment and undergo otoscopy. Cranial nerve assessment and a more complete neurological examination may also be indicated.

External ear

The external ear may easily be damaged by blunt trauma. If bleeding occurs within the subperichondrial space then a haematoma may form. An auricular haematoma should be drained under sterile conditions to prevent infection or fibrosis (Figure 21.3). After aspiration, a compressive dressing is applied to prevent reaccumulation of the haematoma or a seroma. If a haematoma is left untreated then the resulting deformity of the pinna due to loss of cartilage or fibrosis is cosmetically very unsightly forming the classic 'cauliflower ear'.

Lacerations to the pinna should be meticulously closed in layers. The blood supply to this area is so good that healing is rarely a problem. Trauma to the external ear canal is usually due to a laceration caused by instrumentation of the ear canal by cotton buds or other instruments. This can result in severe pain and subsequent infection with debris. Careful cleaning of the canal and the use of antibiotic drops with topical steroids will normally settle the inflammation. Insects will occasionally enter the ear canal and should be killed by instilling warm oil prior to removal with microsuction.

Middle ear

Trauma to the tympanic membrane may occur due to sharp or blunt trauma. A slap to the ear or barotrauma may lead to a tympanic perforation (Figure 21.4). Otoscopy and audiometric testing will demonstrate the extent of the injury. Most traumatic

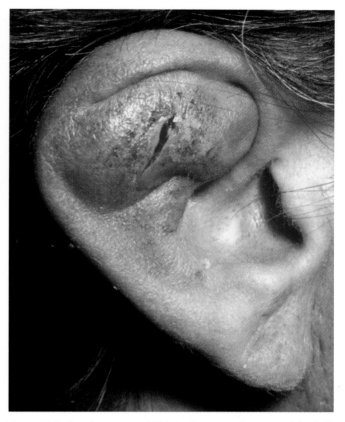

Figure 21.3 Pinna haematoma. (With thanks to my colleague Daniel Hajioff for the use of his clinical photograph of an auricular haematoma.)

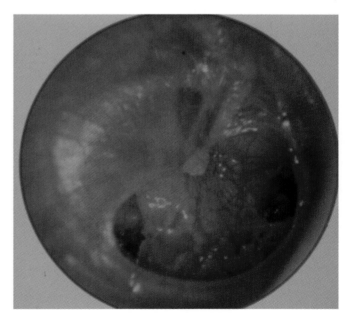

Figure 21.4 Tympanic membrane perforation.

perforations will heal spontaneously but patients should be advised to keep the ear dry until healing has occurred. Welding injuries with a thermal burn to the tympanic membrane are less likely to heal spontaneously. If a perforation persists and is symptomatic a corrective myringoplasty may be performed. Persistent conductive hearing loss after healing should raise the suspicion that the ossicular chain has been damaged.

Barotrauma

Trauma to the middle and inner ear may occur due to a failure to equalise middle ear pressures with the external environment. This may occur during descent in an aircraft or whilst diving. Middle ear haemorrhage and oedema is the most common consequence of such an injury. In these circumstances patients present with discomfort and conductive hearing loss. Spontaneous resolution of symptoms will occur and patients are managed conservatively. In some cases, injury to inner ear structures may occur with sensorineural hearing loss and vertigo. If this occurs then specialist assessment is required urgently.

Temporal bone

Fractures of the temporal bone are divided into longitudinal and transverse fractures (Table 21.1). CT scanning will demonstrate the extent of a temporal bone injury and may demonstrate other injuries such as extradural or subdural haemorrhage. Longitudinal fractures run from the squamous temporal bone, over the roof of the middle ear and along the carotid canal. They are the most common type of fracture (80%). Due to the angle of the fracture the facial nerve and cochlear are not frequently involved. Hearing loss in these cases is usually conductive in nature due to disruption of the ossicles or blood in the middle ear. Any watery discharge from the ear must be collected and tested for the possibility of a CSF leak.

Transverse fractures run across the long axis of the temporal bone and the facial nerve and cochlear are at significant risk of injury. Sensorineural hearing loss is often overlooked as a consequence of head trauma but if persistent may require amplification.

Transverse fractures more commonly cause facial nerve injury with an incidence of facial palsy of 50% in these cases. If a facial palsy develops at the time of injury then the potential recovery of nerve function is greatly reduced and a specialist opinion to consider facial nerve decompression should be sought. Delayed onset or incomplete facial paralysis has a much better outcome. Any patient with a facial palsy should receive advice and attention with regard to protection of the cornea with artificial tears and use of an eye patch at night. If there are no contraindications, steroids may be given to reduce oedema.

Radiation injury

The ear and cochlear are at increasing risk of radiation exposure in modern clinical practice. Current treatment regimens for

malignancies of the head and neck often involve primary or adjuvant radiotherapy and the treatment fields may overlap aural structures. Eustachian tube obstruction may occur leading to a middle ear effusion. This can be treated by placement of a ventilation tube. Cochlear damage with sensorineural hearing loss may occur and may be exacerbated by use of ototoxic chemotherapy treatments. Osteoradionecrosis of the temporal bone has also been reported. It is hoped that newer techniques involving the use of intensity modulated radiotherapy will reduce these risks.

Neck trauma

The complex anatomy and close proximity of vital structures such as major nerves and vessels, airway and digestive tract makes the management of such patients a major diagnostic and therapeutic challenge. The location of trauma in the neck is particularly important and conventionally the neck is demarcated into three zones defined by horizontal planes (Figure 21.5).

Zone I – Clavicle to cricoid cartilage. The base of the neck is vulnerable to injuries to major vascular structures. Penetrating injury may involve the lungs, mediastinum and great vessels.

Zone II – Cricoid cartilage to angle of the mandible. This is the most common zone for injury and assessment and access to injuries is more straightforward due to the location

Zone III – Angle of mandible to base of skull. Assessment and exposure of injury is particularly difficult in this area and special imaging is often required.

Penetrating trauma

Penetrating trauma due to stab wounds or gunshot injury may damage any of the vital structures in the neck (Figure 21.6). Gunshot injuries with high velocity bullets are associated with significant tissue loss and a very high level of morbidity and mortality. Stab wounds may cause injury to underlying structures with minimal evidence of injury superficially. Injury to the cervical spine and spinal cord may also occur and care must be taken to stabilise the spine during assessment and treatment unless injury

Table 21.1 Temporal bone fracture.

	Incidence	Facial nerve injury	CSF leak	Hearing loss
Transverse fracture	20%	50%	Rare	Common: mixed
Longitudinal fracture	80%	20%	Common	Common: conductive

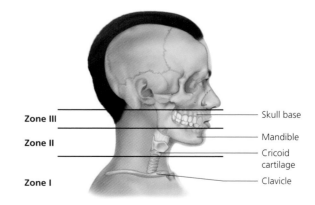

Zone III — Skull base
Zone II — Mandible
— Cricoid cartilage
Zone I — Clavicle

Figure 21.5 The neck is divided into three zones to aid with investigation and treatment of neck trauma.

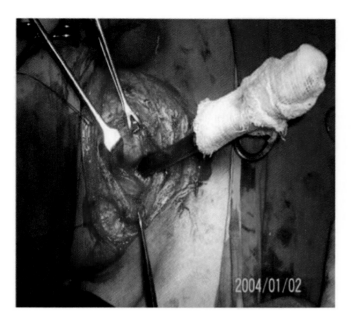

Figure 21.6 Penetrating trauma.

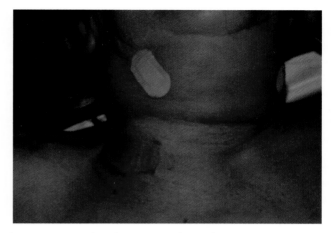

Figure 21.7 Surgical emphysema secondary to blunt trauma.

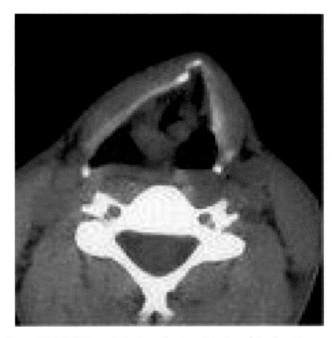

Figure 21.8 A CT Scan illustrating a fracture distortion of the thyroid cartilage (anterior) with moderate soft tissue swelling of the laryngeal soft tissues.

has been excluded. Stabilisation of airway, breathing and circulation must also take place before proceeding with a full assessment.

Vascular and airway injury are a particular issue in these cases. While vascular injury may be evident due to haemorrhage or expanding haematoma, a major vessel may be damaged without immediately being apparent. A high index of suspicion and selective use of imaging by angiography or selective exploration may be required. Any injury penetrating the platysma should arouse suspicion.

Blunt trauma to the neck may occur due to strangulation, hanging or sports injury. The use of seatbelts has reduced the incidence of blunt trauma to the neck during road traffic accidents for car occupants. Pedestrians and cyclists have no such protection and severe blunt tissue injury to the neck region may present.

A rapid and sequential assessment of neck trauma is essential to prevent loss of airway and to avoid the failure to diagnose a serious but masked consequence of the injury.

Airway obstruction may occur due to haemorrhage or secretions in the upper airway. Subcutaneous emphysema, stridor, hoarseness or haemoptysis should lead to a suspicion of airway compromise. If the patient is stable a flexible nasendoscopy may be undertaken to evaluate the airway. CT scanning of the trauma patient should not be undertaken without having first established that the airway is safe. Cricotracheal separation will present with subcutaneous emphysema, aphonia and airway compromise (Figure 21.7).

Intubation after laryngeal trauma may be extremely dangerous if severe endolaryngeal disruption has taken place. Tracheostomy under local anaesthesia is the optimal approach.

In the presence of a suspected traumatised larynx if control of the airway is required. In an emergency situation insufflation with a wide bore cannula inserted into the trachea will improve oxygenation to allow time for an airway to be established.

Blunt trauma to the larynx may result in fracture of the thyroid or cricoid cartilage (Figure 21.8). Severe bruising of the soft tissues

of the larynx may also occur as the larynx is crushed against the cervical spine. Fibreoptic assessment of the larynx is essential to exclude the presence of a haematoma. Undisplaced fractures of the cartilaginous elements of the larynx may be managed conservatively but displaced fractures will normally require open repair and fixation.

The position and state of the vocal cords should be assessed by fibreoptic visualisation. Avulsions of the vocal cord will require repair. Paralysis of the vocal cords due to recurrent laryngeal nerve injury should be recognised and noted.

Pharyngo-oesophageal

Most injuries to the pharynx and oesophagus are caused by penetrating rather than blunt trauma. Patients should be evaluated for dysphagia, haematemesis, odynophagia, surgical emphysema and salivary fistula. A barium swallow will identify approximately 80% of injuries and when combined with rigid oesophagoscopy will identify almost all cases of injury. In the case of small tears, insertion of a nasogastric tube and a policy of keeping the patient nil by mouth will often be sufficient. Significant injury will require exploration and suturing. Delayed recognition of an injury can lead to abscess formation and fistualisation with prolonged morbidity and possible mortality.

Traumatic injury to the oral cavity or oropharynx may occur in children if they fall whilst carrying an item such as a toothbrush or pencil in the mouth. Lacerations to the hard palate can be managed conservatively but injury to the soft palate may merit surgical repair to prevent fistula formation.

Further reading

Atkins BZ, Abbate S, Fisher SR, Vaslef SN. Current management of laryngotracheal trauma: case report and literature review. *J Trauma* 2004;**56**(1):185–90. Review.

Bell RB, Verschueren DS, Dierks EJ. Management of laryngeal trauma. *Oral Maxillofac Surg Clin North Am* 2008;**20**(3):415–30. Review.

Doctor VS, Farwell DG. Gunshot wounds to the head and neck. *Curr Opin Otolaryngol Head Neck Surg* 2007;**15**(4):213–8. Review.

Johnson F, Semaan MT, Megerian CA. Temporal bone fracture: evaluation and management in the modern era. *Otolaryngol Clin North Am* 2008;**41**(3):597–618.

Kesser BW, Chance E, Kleiner D, Young JS. Contemporary management of penetrating neck trauma. *Am Surg* 2009;**75**(1):1–10. Review.

CHAPTER 22

Foreign Bodies

Ricardo Persaud[1], Antony Narula[1] and Patrick J. Bradley[2]

[1]St Mary's Hospital, London, UK
[2]Nottingham University Hospitals, Queen's Medical Centre Campus, Nottingham, UK

OVERVIEW

- The presence of a foreign body is a common occurrence in ENT practice
- Foreign bodies may be organic or inorganic. The former tend to be hydrophilic and therefore will expand over time and should be dealt with promptly
- Sharp objects also require urgent removal, especially if present in the aero-digestive tract
- Miniature batteries wherever lodged or placed – ear, nose or throat MUST be removed immediately, otherwise corrosive injury will follow and this may result in serious complications
- Food bolus without bone may be treated conservatively for 24–48 h with a muscle relaxant, prokinetic agent and analgesia
- Sharp foreign bodies in the throat, tend to lodge in the tonsils, posterior tongue base, valleculae or piriform fossae and may require a general anaesthetic for removal
- Uncooperative children usually require a general anaesthesia for removal of a foreign body within the ear, nose or throat
- Chest X-ray can be normal with an aerodigestive foreign body, so if in doubt it is safer to perform direct endoscopic examination

---

Introduction

The presence of a foreign body in the ear, nose or aerodigestive tract is a common occurrence in ENT practice. It can be a serious and challenging condition associated with considerable morbidity and mortality. Reports from The National Safety Council of America show that foreign bodies in the aerodigestive tract are the most common cause of accidental death in children under 6 years old.

Aural foreign bodies

Aural foreign bodies may present as incidental findings on otoscopy, or with otalgia, otorrhoea and hearing loss. They are most frequent in children under 10 years. Generally, foreign bodies in the ear or elsewhere may be classified as organic (e.g. peanuts, insects) or

ABC of Ear, Nose and Throat, Sixth Edition.
Edited by Harold Ludman and Patrick J. Bradley.
© 2013 John Wiley & Sons, Ltd. Published 2013 by John Wiley & Sons, Ltd.

inorganic (e.g. beads, pins). The former tend to set up an intense inflammatory hydrophilic reaction and therefore must be dealt with promptly. The latter may also require urgent treatment if sharp or a button battery because of the potential to cause significant tissue damage. There is usually no urgency to remove smooth blunt inorganic objects. Insects in the external auditory canal may be drowned instantly with either alcohol or olive oil.

Retrieval

Patients are best managed under the operating microscope in the ENT emergency clinic. Removal is achieved with the use of a Jobson Horne probe, wax hook, suction and/or microforceps. Success is usually accomplished with a raking action. Irrigation should be avoided as organic materials will expand. Blind instrumentation may cause trauma to the canal or tympanic membrane and may impale the foreign material through the eardrum.

Rarely, if a large object is lodged deep in the ear canal, medial to the bony isthmus, or associated with otitis externa, the inflammation may be so severe that the meatus becomes very narrow or closed. Here, a general anaesthetic and a small endaural incision may be required. A general anaesthetic may also be needed to remove aural foreign bodies in young children, who are unable to cooperate.

Nasal foreign bodies

Nasal foreign bodies may present acutely or even after many years. They are most commonly found among 2- to 3-year-old toddlers, impacted between the septum and inferior turbinate and often visible on anterior rhinoscopy.

Organic materials such as tissue paper, sponge or nuts, provoke a profuse inflammatory reaction from the nasal mucosa. Initially the discharge is mucoid but eventually it becomes mucopurulent, and sometimes bloodstained. Inflammation and infection of the sinuses may cause further complications.

Furthermore, a secondary inflammatory response of the nasal vestibular skin (vestibulitis) may develop as a result of the constant discharge. For these reasons, any foul-smelling unilateral nasal discharge in a child, with or without excoriation of the vestibular skin, must be assumed to be due to a foreign body until proven otherwise. This may require examination of both nasal cavities under general anaesthetic.

Retrieval

Foreign bodies, particularly inorganic items, are removed by grasping the object firmly with crocodile forceps or by passing a blunt hook distal to the foreign body and slowly drawing it forward. A microsuction catheter may be used to withdraw objects such as polystyrene beads. Care should be taken not to let the child swallow the object as it is delivered from the nasal cavity. One attempt at removal is usually possible before the child becomes uncooperative. The use of a general anaesthetic may be required.

A battery inserted into the nasal cavity requires urgent examination under general anaesthesia with a good light source, as leakage occurs within hours resulting in corrosive burns and destruction of the nasal septum and inferior turbinate. Corroded mucosa should be irrigated with normal saline and inflamed mucosa treated with Naseptin cream®.

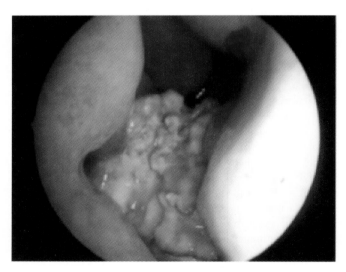

Figure 22.1 A rhinolith in the right nasal cavity.

Late presentation of a nasal foreign body

Occasionally, a small foreign body may lie unnoticed in the nose for many years. Such retained foreign bodies may eventually present with unilateral nasal congestion, epistaxis, discharge and occasionally with sinusitis in late adulthood. Nasal secretions, calcium and magnesium carbonates, and phosphates usually deposit around the foreign body forming a nasal concretion or rhinolith (Figure 22.1), which is demonstrable on CT scan as it is radio-opaque. A rhinolith must be extracted under a general anaesthesia to ensure complete removal and controlled irrigation of the nose.

Orohypopharyngeal foreign bodies

Patients with orohypopharyngeal foreign bodies are usually adults, presenting acutely with pain and drooling. There is often a lateralising pricking sensation and significant odynophagia (pain on swallowing). Pharyngeal foreign bodies are commonly small bones which are not always radio-opaque. Fish bones may lodge in the tonsils, tongue base, valleculae or piriform fossae. Visualisation requires a good light, laryngeal mirror or a flexible nasendoscope. If no foreign body is visible and the patient is well and swallowing, with normal radiography, symptoms may be due to pharyngeal abrasion. The patient should be re-examined after 48 hours and if still symptomatic, should have a CT scan performed to look for a foreign body or signs of an abscess formation. Swallowed or inhaled dentures (especially partial) present special difficulties because their size and configuration compounds impaction and makes removal challenging. The presence of metallic material, such as a metal clasp, on the denture will render it radio-opaque on a plain film radiograph (soft tissue lateral neck is the film of choice) (Figure 22.2). However, most dentures are made from a radiolucent plastic (polymethylmethacrylate) and therefore can be missed easily on such a radiograph. This may delay diagnosis and subsequently lead to life threatening obstruction of aerodigestive tract or erosion of blood vessels. A CT scan would be the investigation of choice if the radiograph appears normal.

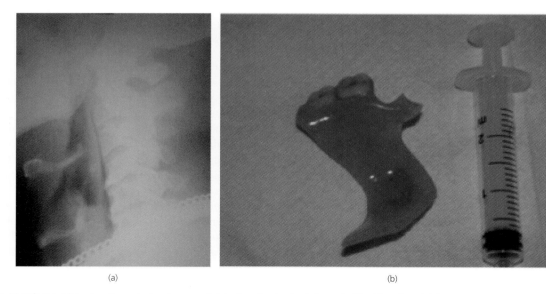

(a) (b)

Figure 22.2 (a) Soft tissue lateral radiograph showing a partial denture foreign body (arrow); (b) retrieved partial denture.

Retrieval

Tonsillar foreign bodies may be removed with a headlight and Tilley's forceps. Tongue base, vallecula and piriform fossa foreign bodies can be removed under local anaesthetic after generous application of topical anaesthetic spray. Indirect laryngoscopy with the patient sitting up, pulling the tongue forward using a swab, allows inspection with a warmed laryngeal mirror, and extraction using a McGill's forceps. Alternatively, the patient may be placed supine with the head below the horizontal in the surgeon's lap. A laryngoscope blade is used to control the tongue and the foreign body is removed under direct vision with a McGill's forceps. The patient should then not eat or drink until the anaesthesia has worn off, at which time he or she may be discharged. On occasions, a lateral soft tissue radiograph of the neck may show a foreign body, such as a coin or fish bone, which will require general anaesthetic removal.

Laryngotracheal foreign bodies

The natural history of a foreign body in the airway or indeed anywhere in the aerodigestive tract, may be divided in the three clinical phases. During the *initial phase* of inhalation the patient may choke, cough, gag or even vomit. This is followed by the *asymptomatic phase* when the foreign body becomes lodged and the reflexes fatigue. This may give a false sense of security that the problem has resolved and lead to a delay in diagnosis. The final *complication phase* may involve erosion, inflammation, infection and abscess formation.

A foreign body in the larynx or trachea may present as an airway emergency which requires urgent first aid (or even an emergency tracheostomy). Large objects that obstruct the glottic inlet may precipitate respiratory arrest. These patients will only survive if resuscitated by an astute paramedic or physician at the scene. There is no time to be assessed and managed by an ENT professional. Small or irregular foreign bodies may produce partial obstruction, but subsequent oedema may compromise the situation. Hoarseness is a common feature of a foreign body in the larynx but other symptoms may mimic croup and lead to a delay in diagnosis and further complications.

Children older than 5 years have been found to be more likely to aspirate objects other than food. Vegetable matter is seen in approximately 70–80% of airway foreign bodies, the most common being peanuts in the USA, watermelon seeds in Egypt and pumpkin seeds in Greece. Plastic pieces comprise 5–15% of airway foreign bodies and tend to remain in the body longer because they are inert and radiolucent. Metallic foreign bodies such as safety pins used to be commonly inhaled or ingested but the prevalence has decreased since the introduction of disposable nappies.

Bronchial foreign bodies

Patients with bronchial foreign bodies typically present with coughing, wheezing and/or reduced breath sounds. The diagnosis may be straightforward when there is a clear history or a witnessed event. However, often it is difficult to make a diagnosis as there are no signs or witnesses. Radiographic imaging may be helpful but frequently there are no positive findings and it may be necessary to review the patient a few days later to see if the symptoms have resolved. It is worth noting that the symptoms of foreign body aspiration may mimic other conditions such as asthma, croup and pneumonia. This can lead to a delay in diagnosis and treatment. Therefore the onset of wheezing in an otherwise healthy child should prompt suspicion of foreign body inhalation, especially if the abnormal breath sound is unilateral. A chest radiograph should be done on all newly diagnosed asthmatics to rule out a foreign body particularly in young children, patients with learning difficulties and psychiatric patients. Within the airway, radiolucent foreign materials should be suspected when there is unexplained atelectasis, unilateral hyperinflation, obstructive emphysema, mediastinal shift or consolidation of the lung on plain X-ray films. Even in the absence of any signs or symptoms but with a good history, a rigid endoscopy under general anaesthesia (Figure 22.3) may be fruitful.

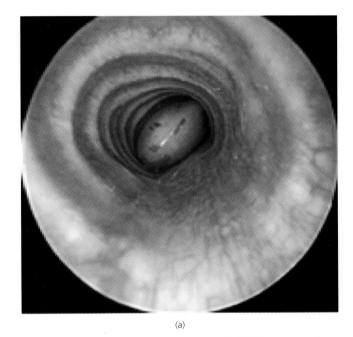

(a)

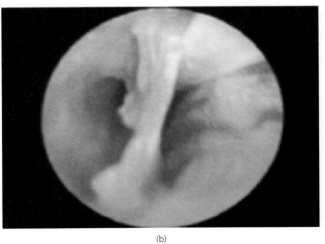

(b)

Figure 22.3 (a) Aspirated kidney bean at the level of the carina; (b) a piece of apple in the right main bronchus.

Bronchial foreign bodies cause three main types of obstruction:

Two-way valve obstruction – Here the foreign body only partially blocks the bronchus and air flows in either direction. Thus the patient may be asymptomatic.

Ball valve obstruction – Here the foreign body obstructs the bronchus completely but allows air to enter distally because of high inspiration pressure. Since expiration is a passive process, the air cannot escape out. This results in hyperinflation of the lung on a chest X-ray (Figure 22.4).

Complete obstruction – Here there is obstruction during both inspiration and expiration, thus leading to atelectasis of the distal segment of the lung.

Retrieval

Any child with respiratory difficulty after an episode of choking following play with small objects should undergo bronchoscopy by an experienced paediatric ENT surgeon and a senior anaesthetist. In adults, objects usually lodge in the right main bronchus, as this is larger and more vertical than the left. In our experience this is not the case children, and we have found equal frequency of airway foreign body in the right and left main bronchi. Any foreign body must be grasped firmly and slowly withdrawn with the appropriate instrument such as optical forceps (Figure 22.5). The

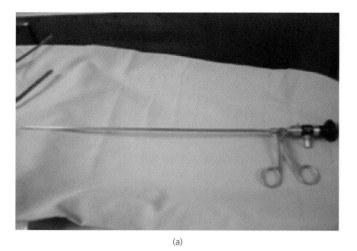

(a)

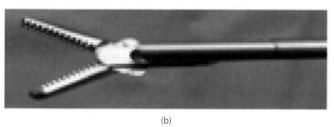

(b)

Figure 22.5 Optical forceps to aid foreign body removal retrieval (a). Open grasper of optical forceps (b).

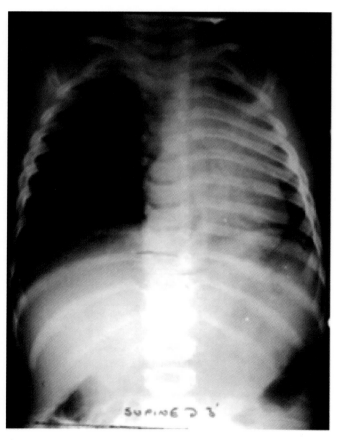

Figure 22.4 Hyperinflated right lung secondary to ball valve obstruction (note mediastinal shift to the left because of air being trapped in the lung).

bronchi are gently cleaned of secretions afterwards by irrigating with some saline.

There may be more than one foreign body, so all areas should be inspected and re-inspected after retrieval. Adults and co-operative children can have bronchial foreign material retrieved under sedation with a flexible bronchoscope. This has an instrument port to allow insertion of flexible forceps, which may be used to extract the material. Rarely, bronchial foreign bodies require thoracotomy by a cardiothoracic surgeon.

It is worth noting that the successful removal of an airway foreign body does not usually have any permanent sequelae. Nevertheless it is important to avoid injury to the tracheal and bronchial mucosa as even a small tear may lead to a pneumothorax or pneumomediastinium when using positive pressure ventilation. Minor bleeding may occur from granulation tissue associated with a chronic foreign body. This may be minimised with the use of topical adrenaline administered via the side port of the ventilating bronchoscope. Antibiotics and physiotherapy may be required to deal with complication such as pneumonia or atelectasis. If there is oedema of the larynx either before or after retrieval of the foreign, a temporary tracheostomy may be needed.

Oesophagus

Adults will usually provide a clear history of swallowing something and can localise approximately where it has impacted. Children, individuals with learning difficulties or psychiatric patients are less able to do so. However, they may present with neck or chest pain, vomiting, excessive salivation, odynophagia and dysphagia, often total. There may also be crepitus, localised tenderness, back pain, fever and tachycardia, if a perforation of the oesophagus is present. Complete obstruction of the oesophagus will cause excessive salivation and regurgitation of any swallowed liquid, including saliva. Some patients may present with haematemesis when a sharp foreign is lodged. Oesophageal foreign bodies may also present with airway obstruction if the trachea is compressed by the impacted object. Occasionally the symptoms are minimal and a longstanding foreign material is discovered when investigating a patient for progressive dysphagia or weight loss.

In children, the commonest object accidentally ingested is a coin (Figure 22.6); meat and vegetable matter impactions are less common compared to adults. In the Asian population, fish bones represent the most commonly encountered foreign body. Round objects, disc battery (Figure 22.7) and sharp object comprise less than 20% of impacted oesophageal foreign bodies.

A food bolus may impact in a normal oesophagus – above the cricopharyngeus, the arch of the aorta, the gastro-oesophageal sphincter – or wherever disease such as stricture or malignancy is present. Soft foreign bodies with no evidence of bone, such as meat boluses, may be managed medically with a muscle relaxant (e.g. buscopan), prokinetic agent (e.g. a macrolide antibiotic such as clarithromycin or erythromycin) and anti-inflammatory drugs. Frequently the bolus may move on over 2 hours. The patient can be reassessed and if drinking normally, can be discharged.

Radio-opaque foreign bodies may be visible on lateral and posteroanterior (PA) radiographs, or there may be an oesophageal air bubble, soft tissue swelling or surgical emphysema. A barium swallow is generally not indicated as the barium makes it difficult to subsequently identify and extract the foreign body. However, Omnipaque™ 500 contrast may be used as it is colourless. In rare cases, an oesophageal foreign body which is not found on initial endoscopy may have migrated extraluminally. Fluoroscopy with contrast or CT scanning may aid in the preoperative localisation. All patients with food bolus impaction should undergo contrast swallow as an outpatient after foreign body retrieval to ensure that there is no local disease to account for the incident.

Retrieval

Removal of a foreign body requires an age specific oesophagoscope which is gently navigated through the cricopharyngeous muscle and carefully advanced until the foreign body is seen. The impacted material is then removed rather than pushed into the stomach. Care must be taken to avoid mucosal damage. A chest X-ray should be performed if there was a traumatic extraction or any concern of significant mucosal tear. In general, close observation of the patient is required after the retrieval of any foreign body. A Gastrografin® contrast swallow may be needed to confirm the diagnosis of a perforation. If a perforation is present, the patient is kept nil by mouth and fed via a nasogastric tube, preferably inserted under radiological guidance, and given a broad spectrum antibiotic intravenously. The contrast swallow is repeated after 7–10 days if the symptoms resolve and there are no signs of infection. If symptoms persist, surgical repair may be necessary.

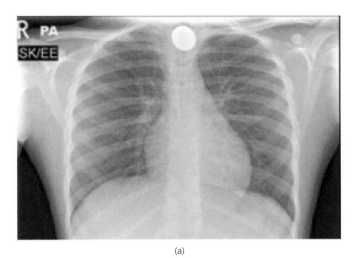

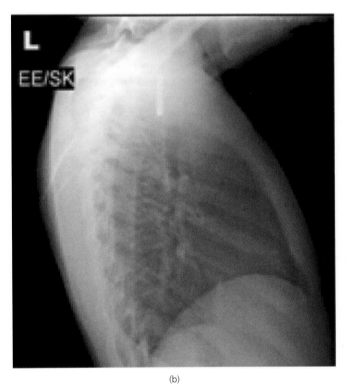

(b)

Figure 22.6 (a) Posteroanterior (PA) and (b) lateral views of a coin in the upper oesophagus at the level of cricopharyngeus.

Close observations with the above management of an oesophageal perforation has resulted in a significant decrease in the mortality rate from 60% to 9%. Following an atraumatic oesophagoscopy, it is usually recommended that the patient be kept nil by mouth for 4 hours as sometimes a paralytic ileus may occur. Sterile water is then introduced, followed by fluids and then a soft diet.

Foreign body prevention

Perhaps the most important way of reducing the incidence of foreign body in the ear, nose and aerodigestive system is raised

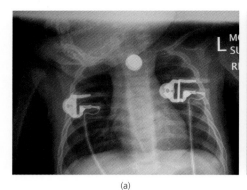

(a)

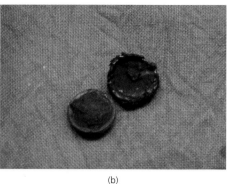

(b)

Figure 22.7 Ingested battery (a) view of impaction in upper oesophagus; (b) when removed.

public awareness. In some countries, many steps have been taken to educate the public, directly or indirectly, of the dangers of small objects in young children. For instance, certain toys are marked unsuitable for specific ages. The Consumer Products Safety Act includes criteria for minimum size of objects allowable for children to play with, but these recommendations are not uniformly enforced. Reiterating to children not to put objects in their mouths could potentially reduce the incidence of aspiration. Children with learning difficulties, oesophageal dysmotility disorders or neurological conditions should be encouraged to chew food slowly and completely to avoid oesophageal impaction or aspiration. However, with the best prevention and will in the world, foreign bodies in the ear, nose and aerodigestive tract will continue to occur.

Conclusions

The incidence of foreign bodies in ENT practice has not changed much over the years, but the safety of the methods used for their retrieval has improved significantly. Foreign bodies in the aerodigestive tract associated with acute symptoms such as coughing, cyanosis, dysphagia or dyspnoea, usually lead to prompt investigation and treatment. However, when the event is unwitnessed or when symptoms are absent, it is difficult to make a diagnosis without having a high index of suspicion. An awareness of the hazards of indwelling prosthesis (such as dentures) by wearers, carers and clinicians is also important to prevent delayed diagnosis. In cases requiring hospital admission, a carefully planned removal of the foreign material under direct vision in a controlled environment is the safest form of management. Successful removal of a foreign body from any location is a very satisfying experience for the entire team involved.

Acknowledgements

With special acknowledgements to Miss Asha Omar for collating the clinical images and proof-reading and Mr Ali Taghi, Miss Catherine Rennie and Mr Raul Cetto for providing the images.

Further reading

Belleza WG, Kalman S. Otolaryngological emergencies in the outpatient setting. *Med Clin Nth Am* 2006;**90**(2):329–53.

Lam HC, Woo JK, van Hasselt CA. Management of ingested foreign bodies: A retrospective review of 5240 patients. *J Laryngol Otol* 2001;**115**:954–7.

Mc Rae D, Premachandra DJ, Gatland DJ. Button batteries in the ear, nose and cervical oesophagus: a destructive foreign body. *J Otolaryngology* 1989; **18**(6):317–19.

Persaud R, Ong C, Sudhakaran N, Bowdler D. (2001) Extraluminal migration of a coin in the oesophagus misdiagnosed as asthma. *Emerg Med J;* **18**: 312–13.

Persaud R, Kapoor L. Foreign Bodies in the Aerodigestive Tract. In: De Souza C,(ed). *Head and Neck Surgery*. Delhi: Jaypee Brothers Medical Publishes Ltd, 2009. pp. 1689–1695.

Hashmi S, Walter J, Smith W, Latis S. Swallowed partial dentures. *J R Soc Med* 2004;**97**(2):72–5.

CHAPTER 23

Neck Swellings

Nick Roland[1] and Patrick J. Bradley[2]

[1]University Hospital Aintree, Liverpool, UK
[2]Nottingham University Hospitals, Queen's Medical Centre Campus, Nottingham, UK

OVERVIEW

- Neck swellings are common findings that present in all age groups from many causes, ranging from congenital to acquired, from cysts, inflammatory, infective to neoplastic disease, encompassing any neck structures

- In the community, the inflammatory lymph node is most common, whereas in hospital thyroid swelling or goitre is most frequently seen

- It behoves all clinicians to understand the embryology and anatomy to aid with making the correct diagnosis thus allowing for appropriate management

- There are more than 100 lymph nodes in each neck, and other organs or glands are singular!

- Knowledge of patient's age, associated symptoms and anatomical location of the lump, is key to proceeding to treatment in General Practice, or is an indication for referral for further investigations, including imaging and surgery

- Neck lumps in adults (over 40 years) should be considered malignant or at least have malignancy excluded by examination of the mucosal surfaces of the head and neck region, and a needle sample of lump be examined by a pathologist

Neck swellings are commonly encountered and present at all ages. The differential diagnosis of a neck mass is extensive. In the community inflammatory lymph nodes are most common, while in the hospital environment the thyroid swelling or goiter is most frequently seen. It therefore behoves all clinicians to understand the embryology and anatomy to aid with making the correct diagnosis and following an appropriate management algorithm.

Anatomy of the normal neck

The old surgical aphorism,

consider the anatomical structures and then the pathology that can arise from these

is never more appropriate than when one contemplates the causes of a lump in the neck.

Clinicians are taught to examine a patients' neck, its landmarks and contents, early in their undergraduate careers, and for the remainder of their clinical life should never have to reconsider what they have been taught. Patients are untaught, and hence when they get a symptom located to their neck, naturally palpate their own neck and that of others, and consider possible diseases diagnoses and become alarmed with what they can feel!

The normal glandular structures are consistent in their location; the thyroid gland is a bilobed structure located along the midline of the neck on either side of the trachea, above the sternal notch, and below the cricoid cartilage. The parotid gland is found in front of the ear or pinna, and extends from the cheek bone (zygoma) above, down and behind to the mastoid tip, below into the upper neck near the hyoid bone and forward onto the cheek for about 2–3 cms. The submandibular gland, is, located below the posterior half of the mandible, but not extending beyond the angle of the mandible, above the hyoid bone (Figure 23.1) (see Chapter 1).

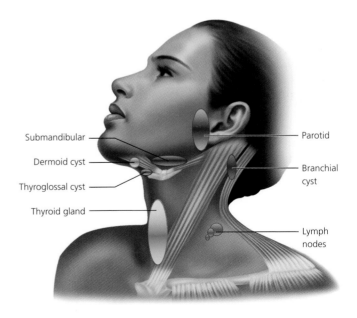

Submandibular — Parotid
Dermoid cyst — Branchial cyst
Thyroglossal cyst —
Thyroid gland — Lymph nodes

Figure 23.1 Common neck lumps.

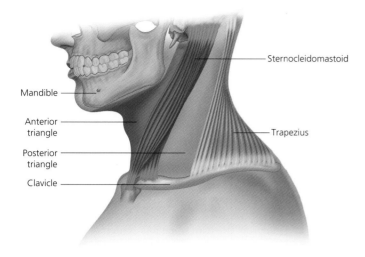

Figure 23.2 The lateral neck. Anterior triangle is bounded posteriorly by the posterior border of the SCM muscle, and the posterior triangle is between the posterior border of the SCM and the anterior border of the trapezius muscle and the clavicle inferiorly.

Within each side of the neck there are located more than 100 lymph nodes, usually impalpable, and distributed mainly along the jugular chain, to be found within each of the 5 clinically and anatomically described levels in the anterior neck and in the single but divided level in the posterior neck. The posterior border of the SCM muscle separates the anterior neck from the posterior neck (Figure 23.2). While there are other major structures within the neck, such as nerves, blood vessels, muscles, cartilages and bones, knowledge of their anatomic outline should allow the examiner to consider any such abnormal enlargement or swellings in certain anatomic locations to be included within a differential diagnosis.

Reaching a diagnosis

Reaching a diagnosis obviously requires some knowledge of the potential pathology. It is difficult to present an exhaustive list of the potential causes of a neck swelling, but a simple classification is tabulated below (Box 23.1).

> **Box 23.1 More common causes of neck swellings**
>
> - **Congenital**: lymphangiomas, dermoids, thyroglossal cysts
> - **Developmental**: branchial cysts, laryngoceles, pharyngeal pouches
> - **Skin and subcutaneous tissue**: sebaceous cyst, lipoma
> - **Thyroid swellings**: multinodular goitre, solitary thyroid nodule
> - **Salivary gland tumours**: pleomorphic adenoma, Warthins tumour
> - **Tumours of the parapharyngeal space**: deep lobe parotid, chemodectoma
> - **Reactive neck lymphadenopathy**: tonsillitis, glandular fever, HIV
> - **Malignant neck node**: carcinoma metastases (unknown primary), lymphoma

In practical terms, the diagnosis is reached from the patients' age, the history, location and physical examination of the neck (Box 23.2), followed by a thorough examination of the upper aerodigestive tract and the results of appropriate tests and investigations.

> **Box 23.2 Reaching a diagnosis**
>
> - Age
> - History
> - Location
> - Examination of the lump
> - Examination of the head and neck

Age

The first consideration should be the patient's age group (Table 23.1). In general, neck masses in children and young adults are more commonly inflammatory than congenital and only occasionally neoplastic. However, the first consideration in the older adult should be that the mass is neoplastic. The "rule of 80" is often applied as a useful guide. In adults 80% of non-thyroid neck masses are probably neoplastic and 80% of these masses are malignant. This statement probably refers to masses over 2 cm in diameter, in patients over 35 years of age, and for clinicians who are not regularly seeing patients with neck masses. A neck mass in a child, on the other hand, has a 90% probability of being a benign condition of which 55% are congenital.

History

Onset and duration of symptoms is one of the most important historical points. Inflammatory disorders are usually acute in onset and resolve within 2–6 weeks. Cervical lymphadenitis is often associated with a recent upper respiratory tract infection. In contrast, congenital masses are often present since birth as a small, asymptomatic mass which enlarges rapidly after a mild upper respiratory tract infection. Metastatic carcinoma tends to have a short history with progressive enlargement. Transient post-prandial (after meals) swelling in the submandibular or parotid area is suggestive

Table 23.1 Age in relation to possible diagnoses.

	Child (0–15 years)	Young adult (16–35 years)	Adult (35 years +)
Congenital	Cystic hygroma Thyroglossal duct cyst	Branchial cyst	Very uncommon
Inflammatory	Very common	Less common	Rare
Salivary disease	Inflammatory	Sialolithiasis	Neoplasms
Thyroid disease	Uncommon Malignancy	Usually endocrine Papillary carcinoma	Most often endocrine Thyroid malignancy
Neoplasms	Rare	Lymphoma Metastases	Lymphoma Squamous cell carcinoma Metastases

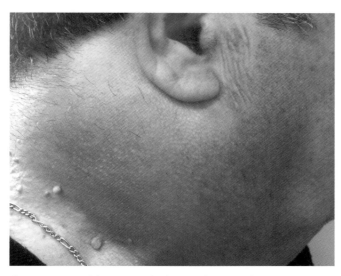

Figure 23.3 An adult patient with a large neck mass with systemic symptoms – proven lymphoma.

Table 23.2 Examination checklist.

	Lymphadenitis	Branchial cyst	Goitre	Dermoid cyst	Thyroglossal cyst
Painful?	Yes	Possible	Possible	Possible	Seldom
Associated symptoms?	Yes	No	Yes	No	No
Moves with swallowing?	No	No	Yes	No	Yes
Midline?	Uncommonly	No	No	Yes	Yes
Moves on protruding the tongue?	No	No	No	No	Yes

of salivary gland duct obstruction – a stone or a stenosis. Bilateral diffuse tender parotid enlargement is suggestive of parotitis, most commonly mumps, usually school children, and manifests in local epidemics and can only get the disease once!

One must also be mindful that associated symptoms both specifically to the mass and symptoms suggestive of a systemic process such as fever, night sweats, fatigue or weight loss (consider lymphoma) must be sought and documented (Figure 23.3). Symptoms of sore throat or upper respiratory tract infection may suggest an inflammatory cervical lymphadenopathy. Persistent hoarseness or sore throat, pain on swallowing, cough and sensation of a lump in the throat are risk symptoms of an upper aerodigestive tract malignancy. The symptoms are particularly relevant in patients who are over the age of 40 years and smoke cigarettes. These are the patients who should be referred via the 'Two week proforma' to the local ENT service.

Location

While congenital and organ masses are more consistent in their locations, metastatic nodes follow a predictive pattern and help in identifying the primary malignancies (see Chapter 1).

Examination

A full head and neck examination (see Chapter 1) including mucosal surfaces is important, especially when suspecting malignancies (Table 23.2).

Congenital masses may be tender when infected or inflamed, but are generally soft, smooth and mobile. A tender, mobile mass or a high suspicion of inflammatory adenopathy with an otherwise negative examination may warrant a clinical trial of a broad-spectrum antibiotic and a review after 2 weeks. Chronic inflammatory masses and lymphomas are often non-tender and rubbery and may be mobile or feel like a "matted mass" of nodules. In older age groups, the submandibular and parotid glands may become ptotic (droopy) and mimic a neck mass, and can cause concern to patients.

Diagnostic studies

- Full blood count and ESR.
- Viral serology: Epstein–Barr Virus, cytomegalovirus and toxoplasmosis.
- Throat swab: occasionally helpful (but must be sent immediately in the proper medium).
- Thyroid function tests and ultrasound in all cases of thyroid enlargement.
- Chest X-ray in smokers with persistent neck lump.
- Ultrasound scan (USS) can delineate the position, size, and sometimes the nature of a neck lump. It may delineate impalpable nodes and thyroid nodules. The shape of a lymph node (normally oval with a fatty hilum) can be altered by malignant disease (round shape with irregular margins and altered hilum). Although USS is performed with a view to guiding a fine needle aspiration biopsy (USSgFNAB) it should be noted that a biopsy may not be indicated if the size and nature of the lump is obviously benign.
- Fine needle aspiration biopsy (FNAB) is helpful for the diagnosis for neck masses and is indicated in any neck mass that is not an obvious abscess and persists following prescribed antibiotic therapies. A negative result may require a repeat FNAB, USSgFNAB or even an open biopsy, correlating with other clinical information.
- Radionucleotide scanning: for suspected parathyroid and thyroid gland masses.
- Computed Tomography (CT) scanning can distinguish cystic from solid lesions, define the origin and full extent of deep, ill-defined masses, and when used with contrast can delineate vascularity or blood flow.
- Magnetic Resonance Imaging (MRI) is useful for parapharyngeal and skull base masses and for assessment for unknown primary carcinomas. With contrast it is good for vascular delineation and MRI angiography may substitute for arteriography in the pulsatile mass or mass with a bruit or thrill.

See Table 23.3 for differential diagnosis according to position.

Benign neck lesions

Haemangiomas and lymphangiomas

These are congenital lesions usually presenting within the first year of life. Lymphangiomas usually remain unchanged into adulthood, whereas haemangiomas often resolve spontaneously within the first decade (Figure 23.4). A lymphangioma mass is soft, doughy,

Table 23.3 Differential diagnosis according to position.

Midline lumps	Dermoid cysts
	Thyroglossal cyst (moves on protruding lump)
	Thyroid lump (moves on swallowing)
	Lymphadenopathy

Lateral neck lumps	
Submandibular triangle	Reactive lymphadenopathy (younger age group)
	Neoplastic lymphadenopathy (firm, non-tender, older age group)
	Submandibular gland disease (sialadenitis, sialolithiasis, neoplasm)
Anterior triangle	Reactive lymphadenopathy or lymphoma (younger age group)
	Specific infective adenopathy (TB, HIV toxoplasmosis, actinomycosis)
	Neoplastic lymph adenopathy (firm, non-tender, lymphoma or squamous cell carcinoma)
	Branchial cyst (2nd-3rd decades)
	Thyroid masses (toxic goitre, cyst, neoplasm: benign or malignant)
	Parotid gland disease (sialadenitis, cysts, sialolithiasis, neoplasm)
	Paraganglioma (carotid body tumor, glomus vagale)
	Laryngocoele (enlarges with blowing)
	Cystic hygroma/lymphangioma
Posterior triangle	Reactive lymphadenopathy (younger age group)
	Neoplastic lymph adenopathy (firm, non-tender, older age group)
	Lipoma
	Cervical rib

controversial, but should be given until the expected proliferative phase has elapsed.

Sebaceous cysts

These are common masses presenting in older patients. They are slow growing, but may become fluctuant and painful when infected. Diagnosis is made clinically; the overlying skin is adherent to the underlying mass and a punctum is often seen. Excisional biopsy confirms the diagnosis and is curative.

Lipoma

Lipomas or fatty lumps are the most common benign soft tissue tumour in the neck (Figure 23.5). They present as a poorly defined, soft mass usually presenting after the fourth decade. They are usually asymptomatic, soft to touch and deep to the skin. Occasionally they

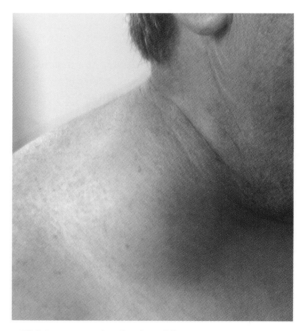

Figure 23.5 Lower posterior triangle neck lipoma.

ill-defined, and may present with pressure effects. Haemangiomas often appear bluish on the overlying skin and are compressible. CT or MRI may help define the extent of the neoplasm, especially when involving the airway. Treatment of lymphangioma includes injection of picibanil or excision. For haemangiomas, treatment is generally non-surgical and to await spontaneous resolution. The aggressive proliferative types are treated using propranolol +/− steroids orally, but this must be given under specialist hospital care because of its side-effects. The duration of treatment remains

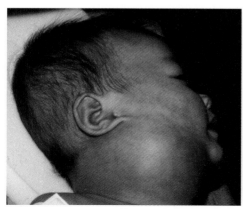

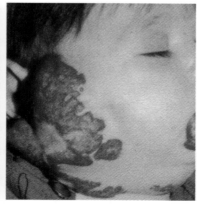

(a)

(b)

Figure 23.4 Congenital neck masses in children: (a) lymphangioma; (b) haemangiomas. (Courtesy of Dr T. McGill, Boston, USA)

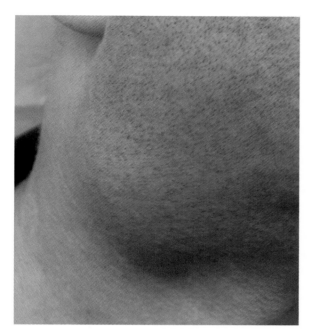

Figure 23.6 Branchial cyst in young patient.

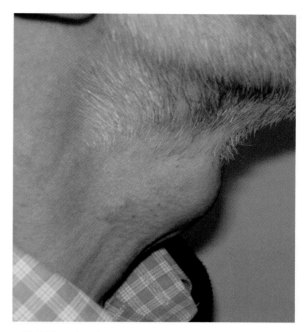

Figure 23.7 Thyroglossal cyst.

can grow very large and be deeply seated between muscles and nerves. FNAC or MRI scan will confirm the diagnosis and extent of the lesion. Surgery is generally for cosmetic reasons, but may be indicated when there appears to increasing in size or doubt about the accuracy of diagnosis.

Branchial cleft cyst

Most often presents in young adults following an upper respiratory tract infection, as a sudden onset of a tender oval mass, which is described as being 4–6 cms in size, located in the upper neck, junction of upper and middle third anterior border of the SCM muscle (Figure 23.6). If presentation is as an acute infected process then the lesion should be treated with antibiotics followed by elective interval surgery. The differential diagnosis is between a solid mass – most likely to be a lymphoma in this age group. In patients over 40 years of age, there is a possibility that such a presentation could represent a cystic metastasis from a papillary thyroid carcinoma or a cystic metastasis from a primary pharyngeal squamous cell carcinoma. Treatment is surgical excision of the mass with histological confirmation of the true nature of the cystic process.

Thyroglossal duct cyst

This is a common congenital midline neck mass, but it may lay off-centre at the lateral edge of the thyroid cartilage (Figure 23.7). On occasions it can be found along a tract from the hyoid bone to the anterior mediastinum. The lesion elevates on tongue protrusion as it is attached to the hyoid bone. This movement distinguishes a thyroglossal cyst from a dermoid cyst or an enlarged lymph node. Should presentation be as an infected cyst then treatment should be with board-spectrum antibiotic followed by interval surgery. Surgery must include excising the mid-portion of the hyoid bone (Sistrunk's procedure) as not to do so is likely to result

in incomplete excision resulting in a discharging thyroglossal fistula. This will require to be treated subsequently by further surgery.

Inflammatory cervical adenitis

Benign cervical adenopathy is the most common cause of a neck mass in children. Palpable nodes are present in 40% of infants and approximately 55% of children. Thus all paediatric age groups have lymph nodes that are palpable but not necessarily associated with an underlying systemic infection or illness. Cervical lymph nodes that are asymptomatic and <1 cm in diameter may be considered normal in children under 12 years of age. Lymphadenitis in children may have a viral, bacterial, fungal, parasitic or non-infectious aetiology. The most common cause of bacterial cervical adenitis in children is staphylococcus aureus and Group A streptococci. Anaerobic bacteria also may be involved. Suspected cases of bacterial adenitis will usually respond to a 10 day course of a beta-lactamase- resistant agent, with complete resolution of the mass in 4–6 weeks. However in cases of progressive symptoms, enlargement of nodes, or the development of fluctuation or an abscess, aspiration or incision and drainage should be performed and the pus sent for culture.

Granulomatous cervical adenitis

This is another common cause of infectious cervical adenitis in children. Aetiology may be tuberculous or non-tuberculous mycobacteria. Atypical or non-tuberculous mycobcateria are the most common causes arising from Mycobacterium avium-intracellulare, or Mycobacterium scrofulacerum. Typically the skin overlying the involved area undergoes violaceous colour change, with skin breakdown and drainage (Figure 23.8). Surgery using complete nodal excision is the preferred treatment, but when involving areas such as the parotid gland curettage has been equally effective, all cases should have post-operative clarithomycin.

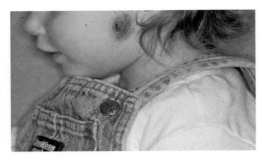

Figure 23.8 Atypical mycobaceria in the parotid area in a child. (Courtesy of Dr T. McGill, Boston, USA)

In general, if a presumed cervical adenopathy mass does not respond to conventional antibiotics, located in the supraclavicular fossa, or posterior triangle, or accompanied by other symptoms such as pain, fever or weight loss, a biopsy should be performed after a complete head and neck work-up to rule out malignancy or granulomatous disease. The rule of thumb is if the neck mass in an infant or child is bigger than a "golf-ball" after 3–4 weeks of observation or a "course of antibiotics", then a serious underlying disease needs to be excluded – lymphoma or sarcoma (Figure 23.9a and b).

Salivary gland enlargement

Salivary gland enlargement is the common denominator of systemic metabolic, endocrine and autoimmune disorders. Diseases such as obesity, starvation, diabetes and hypothyroidism are associated with fatty infiltration of the salivary glands most noticeable in the parotid glands. Of course the commonest cause of parotid enlargement seen in the community is viral sialadenitis which can be caused by a variety of viruses: coxsackie virus A, echoviruses, influenza A, cytomegalovirus and most commonly the mumps (paramyxovirus). Mumps is usually a self limiting disease requiring supportive measures and pain relief. Other causes include sialadenitis or stone formation which can block the duct and present as a swelling of the major glands – parotid and submandibular gland.

Salivary gland enlargement due to neoplasms accounts for < 5% in children. The most common benign tumour of the salivary glands in children is the haemangioma, followed by pleomorphic adenoma and lymphangiomas. Benign pleomorphic adenoma is treated similarly as in adults, with FNAC to confirm the diagnosis followed by complete surgical excision. In adults pleomorphic adenoma and adenolymphoma (Warthin's Tumour) are the commonest tumours (Figure 23.10). Salivary gland malignancy in children is uncommon and usually presents in children over 10 years of age. The most common malignant salivary gland tumours in children and adults are the mucoepidermoid carcinoma, followed by acinic cell carcinoma and adenoid cystic carcinoma. Diagnosis is by FNAC, evaluation by CT scan and treatment is by surgery excision, with or without post-operative radiotherapy.

Thyroid masses

Thyroid neoplasms are a common cause of anterior compartment neck masses in all age groups with a female predominance and are mostly benign (Figure 23.11). All children with a thyroid swelling or mass should be investigated for the possibility of a malignancy.

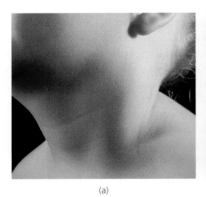

(a)

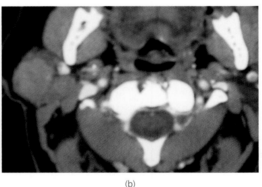

(b)

Figure 23.9 Cervical adenopathy: (a) mass in upper neck; (b) CT scan of neck mass – proven diagnosis lymphoma.

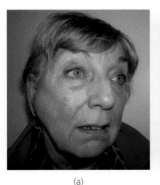

(a)

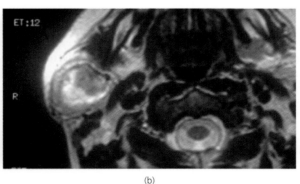

(b)

Figure 23.10 Parotid mass: (a) pre- and infra-auricular area, painless; (b) CT imaging – proven a pleomorphic adenoma.

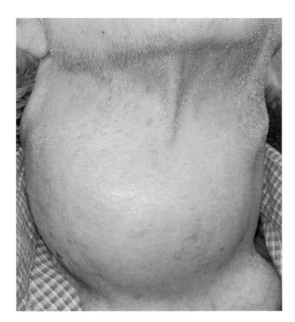

Figure 23.11 Anaplastic thyroid mass.

Fine-needle aspiration of thyroid masses has become the standard of care and ultrasound may help to determine if the mass is cystic or solid. Unsatisfactory aspirates should be repeated, and negative aspirates should be followed up with a repeat FNAC and examination in 3 months time.

Paraganglioma (carotid body tumour, glomus vagale)

These are rare tumours usually found in adults (Figure 23.12). They are slow growing painless lumps which have an average presentation at the fifth decade. Sometimes they present as a parapharyngeal mass pushing the tonsil medially and anteriorly or as a firm mass in the anterior triangle of the neck. Biopsy is contraindicated and MRI angiography is the investigation of choice. Surgical removal is based on patient factors and presenting symptoms.

Malignant neck masses

The incidence of neoplastic cervical lymphadenopathy increases with age and approximately 75% of lateral neck masses in patients older than 40 years are caused by malignant tumours. In a large reported series from the UK it was reported that 74% of enlarged cervical nodes had developed from head and neck primary sites and only 11% had come from primary sites outside that region. The finding of a mass in the left supraclavicular fossa also called a Virchow's node maybe an indication of an infraclavicular metastatic malignancy – most commonly an upper GIT, lung of GUT system (Figure 23.13).

Thorough examination of the upper aerodigestive tract (to include the oral cavity, postnasal space, pharynx and larynx) and the thyroid gland is therefore mandatory.

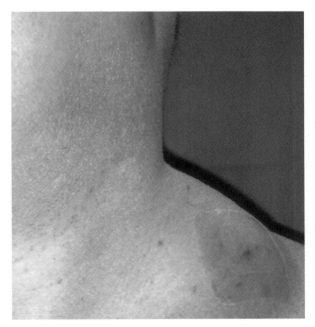

Figure 23.13 A supraclavicular mass.

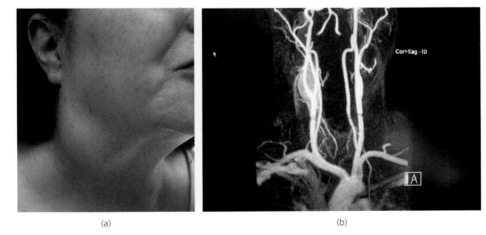

(a)   (b)

Figure 23.12 Carotid body tumour (paragangliomas): (a) clinical picture; (b) angiography.

Primary of Unknown Origin is a term is applied to patients with a metastatic carcinoma in cervical lymph nodes with an "occult primary". A careful search will usually reveal the primary tumour in the skin or mucosal surfaces of the head and neck, or rarely, in an area below the clavicles, such as the lungs. It is important to thoroughly search for the primary tumour by all available diagnostic methods. A thorough history and endoscopic examination will reveal most cases, but imaging (MRI and PET CT) and panendoscopy with selective targeted biopsies from high risk sites (nasopharynx, ipsilateral tonsil excision, base of tongue and piriform fossa) may be required. In approximately 3–11% of cases the primary tumour remains elusive and it is these that the term "primary of unknown origin" should be reserved.

Indications for specialist referrals

In the primary care setting, neck lumps are mostly caused by inflammatory conditions that are self limiting, resolving within 2–6 weeks. A course of appropriate antibiotics with a 2-week follow-up assessment is an appropriate first line of management. Failure to resolve requires hospital referral, especially if any presenting signs or symptoms suggest a possible underlying malignancy. In a high risk patient for malignancy with a neck lump, immediate referral is recommended, usually adults who have a history of smoking or chewing tobacco and indulging in excessive drinking of alcohol. Lumps associated with weight loss or dysphonia (hoarseness), dysphagia (swallowing), or dyspnoea (breathing) for 3 weeks or more should be referred urgently for a head and neck assessment.

Further reading

Addams-Williams J, Watkins D, *et al*. Non-thyroid neck lumps appraisal of the role of fine needle aspiration cytology. *Eur Arch Otorhinolaryngol* 2009;**266**(3):411–15.

Cozens N. A systematic review that involves one-stop neck lumps clinics. *Clin Otolaryngol* 2009;**34**(1):6–11.

Frazer L, Moore P, Kubba H. Atypical mycobacterial infection of the head and neck in children: a 5 year retrospective review. *Otolaryngol Head Neck Surg* 2008;**138**(3):311–14.

Jones AS, Cook JA, Phillips D, Roland NJ. Squamous carcinoma presenting as an enlarged cervical lymph node. *Cancer* 1993;**72**:1756–61.

MacGregor FB, Mc Allister KA. Neck lumps and head and neck tumors in children. *Br J Hosp Med* 2008;**69**(4):205–10. Review.

Mahoney EJ, Spiegel JH. Evaluation and management of malignant cervical lymphadenopathy with an unknown primary tumor. *Otolaryngol Clin North Am* 2005;**38**(1):87–97.

Roland NJ, Fenton J & Bhalla R. Management of a lump in the neck. *Hospital Med* 2002;**4**:205–9.

CHAPTER 24

Head and Neck Cancer

Patrick J. Bradley

Nottingham University Hospitals, Queen's Medical Centre Campus, Nottingham, UK

Definition

Head and neck cancer encompasses any malignant diagnosis of organs and supporting tissues, the majority being the mucous membrane, above the clavicle, yet not including the brain and orbits. Skin cancer is generally not included, yet some clinicians will also manage such patients, as both diseases occur in a similar aged population. Thus cancers of the oral cavity, nose, paranasal sinuses and nasopharynx, oropharynx, larynx and hypopharynx are included (Figure 24.1). Also included, but may vary worldwide, are the salivary glands and the thyroid.

The majority of head and neck cancers are squamous cell carcinomas of the oral cavity and larynx, whereas cancers of the salivary glands and the thyroid gland are unique to their anatomical area. When cancer affects the head and neck area major functions can be affected such as speech, voice, swallowing, taste, and smell, and treatment can result in additional functional alterations resulting

ABC of Ear, Nose and Throat, Sixth Edition.
Edited by Harold Ludman and Patrick J. Bradley.
© 2013 John Wiley & Sons, Ltd. Published 2013 by John Wiley & Sons, Ltd.

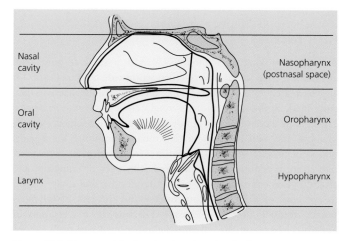

Figure 24.1 Diagram of the head and neck anatomic sites.

in variable effects on patient's quality of life. When making a treatment decision a balance between the efficiency of treatment and the likelihood of survival needs to be considered, including functional and quality of life outcomes. Attempts to encompass such decision-making has resulted in the "Head and neck cancer multidisciplinary team (MDT)" meeting weekly to discuss and plan patients treatment, anticipate any physical and psychological support required, and to plan functional rehabilitation.

Incidence

Cancer of the mouth is the tenth most common cancer worldwide, but is the seventh most common cause of cancer deaths. Nasopharyngeal cancer is largely restricted to southern China, and oral cavity cancer is highest in India. The highest incidence of head and neck cancer is seen in South East Asia, Western Pacific and Western Europe. The male to female ratio reported varies from 2:1 to 15:1 depending on the site of disease.

Head and neck cancer in the European Union (EU) 2008, reports that laryngeal cancer is the most frequent diagnosed, most often within the age 50–70 years and is rarely made in patients younger than 40 years. The overall incidence of laryngeal cancer was 3.4 per 100 000 with a mortality of 1.6. The incidence in men is 6.8, with a mortality of 3.4, and the incidence in women is 0.6, with a mortality

Table 24.1 Recorded numbers of new cases of head and neck cancer in the UK 2004.

Site	England Men/Women	Wales Men/Women	Scotland Men/Women	N.Ireland Men/Women	UK Men/Women
Oral	2441/1299	189/81	430/200	89/40	3149/1620
Larynx	1424/269	91/24	234/71	40/13	1789/377
Nasopharynx	128/59	4/2	9/5	10/0	151/66
Salivary gland	260/201	19/13	22/16	6/8	307/238
Thyroid gland	373/1002	25/55	41/112	6/27	445/1196
Total	7456	503	1140	239	9338

of 0.2 per 100 000. The estimated incidence per 100 000 of laryngeal cancer ranges from 8.9 in Hungary to 1.6 in Sweden, with men more likely to be affected 5–7:1 women. The recorded new cases by country, sex and site in the UK are tabulated (Table 24.1).

Risk factors

Tobacco (smoking and smokeless products such as quid) and alcohol are the major risk factors worldwide and account for approximately 75% of all cases. Their effects are multiplicative when combined. Smoking is more strongly associated with laryngeal cancer and alcohol consumption than it is with cancers of the pharynx and oral cavity. Quitting tobacco smoking for a short period of time (1–4 years) results in a head and neck cancer risk reduction of around 30% compared with current smoking, and after 20 years can reduce the risk of developing oral cavity cancer to the level of a lifelong non-smoker and the risk of laryngeal cancer by 60% after 10–15 years. The benefits of cessation or quitting alcohol, on the risk of developing head and neck cancer, are observed after more than 20 years, when the level of risk reaches that of non-drinkers. While most people who smoke and drink do not develop a head and neck cancer, a genetic predisposition has been demonstrated. Virus infections as a risk factor have been recognised since the mid 1960s with Epstein–Barr virus (EBV) and the development of nasopharyngeal cancer. Recently the HPV subtype16 (human papilloma virus) has been associated with a significant rise in the diagnosis of oropharyngeal cancer. This disease is a distinct disease entity, with patients being diagnosed younger (usually under 50 years), usually not indulging in smoking and excess alcohol intake, most often presenting with enlarging and palpable cervical lymph nodes.

Presentation

Patients with head and neck cancers present with a variety of symptoms, depending on its site location. Laryngeal cancer commonly presents with hoarseness. Pharyngeal cancer may present in the early phase with a sore throat, local pain, "feeling of a lump in the throat" or a neck mass, and when late with dysphagia, hoarseness and/or breathing difficulty. Oral cavity cancer presents early with a painful ulcerative lesion on the lateral border of the tongue with/or without a neck swelling (Figure 24.2). Nose tumours may present with unilateral nasal obstruction, a bloody nasal discharge or even deafness in one ear!

Patients with a head and neck cancer present frequently with a neck swelling which is gradually increasing in size. Many others are

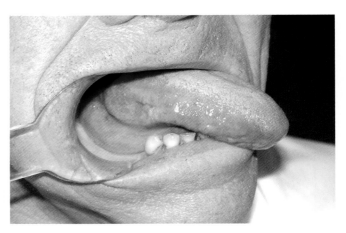

Figure 24.2 Squamous cell carcinoma on the lateral border of tongue.

diagnosed with non-specific symptoms commonly associated with benign conditions, such as throat discomfort, earache, cough or alteration to voice quality. Within the NHS, "Referral guidelines for the patients with suspected cancer" have been drawn up (Box 24.1)

Box 24.1 Referral guidelines for the patients with suspected cancer

Head and neck: urgent referral

- An unexplained lump in the neck, of recent onset, or a previously undiagnosed lump that has changed over a period of 3–6 weeks
- An unexplained persistent swelling of the parotid or submandibular gland
- An unexplained persistent sore or painful throat
- Unilateral unexplained pain in the head and neck area for >4 weeks, associated with otalgia (ear ache) but a normal otoscopy
- Unexplained ulceration of the oral mucosa or mass persisting for >3 weeks
- Unexplained red or white patches (including suspected lichen planus) of the oral mucosa that are painful or swollen or bleeding

Thyroid: urgent referral

- A solitary nodule increasing in size
- A history of neck irradiation
- A family history of an endocrine tumour
- Unexplained hoarseness or voice change
- Cervical lymphadenectomy
- Very young (prepubertal) patient
- Patient aged 65 years or older

and patients with such symptoms will be seen by a cancer specialist within the "2-week rule".

What's the hospital process?

Patients who are referred with "suspicious symptoms" or who have been referred for other causes, are processed in a similar manner – a history is taken of present symptoms, past diseases, medications and hospital admissions. Patients may have head and neck symptoms related to other cancers, i.e. lymphoma, oesophageal or lung cancer. All patients are examined and investigated in a similar fashion.

Should the primary site of malignancy not be detected then recent advanced in diagnostic imaging have helped greatly by using a technique of fusion positive emission tomography and computerised tomography, which used a labelled isotope 18F fluorodeoxyglucose (18F-FDG) which is taken up preferentially by any cells that have a high metabolic activity, at the time of the test, and cancer cells are one such area of activity. This technique has not only a role in the diagnosis of patients with "the occult primary", but can detect locoregional evidence of metastatic disease. It can also be used on completion of treatment to evaluate response, potentially identify at an early stage persistent disease and allow for alternative treatment regimens to be considered.

Other tests may be performed as indicated and include performing immune-histochemistry on the biopsy specimen for viruses such as EBV and HPV.

Prognostic factors

Site and TNM

The most important prognostic factors are site of the primary disease and its TNM stage (T, tumour; N, nodal status; M, metastases). The TNM staging system has been unified worldwide and divides the disease stages into early and late (Table 24.2). The T stage defines the size or "bulk" of the primary tumour, the N stage defines the presence or absence of cervical nodal involvement and the extent of involvement, and the M stage is the absence or presence of distant metastasis. Staging of patients can only be completed when "all information" is available, including a written histology confirming the pathological diagnosis.

Table 24.2 Stage groupings.

Stage I	T1	N0	M0	Early Disease
Stage II	T2	N0	M0	
Stage III	T1 T2	N1	M0	Early Advanced
	T3	N0 N1	M0	
Stage IVA	T1 T2 T3	N2	M0	Advanced Resectable
	T4a	N0 N1 N2	M0	
Stage IVB	Any T	N3	M0	Advanced Unresectable
	T4b	Any N	M0	
Stage IVC	Any T	Any N	M1	Advanced Metastatic

T, tumour; N, nodal status; M, metastases; Stage I & II – Early Disease, Stage III & IV – Advanced Disease.

Co-morbidity

Co-morbidity is the presence of illness unrelated to the tumour. Its presence affects prognosis in head and neck cancer patients, and is contributed to tobacco, alcohol and substance abuse. The effects are associated with increased mortality especially in the early years after treatment and a greater impact on the younger patients, modification of treatment options resulting in an adverse influence on disease specific survival, higher incidence of and more severe complications, adverse impact on quality of life and increased cost of treatment.

Treatment

Modern management of patients with cancer, and none more so than head and neck cancer is by clinical specialists whose major daily working interest is cancer. Such clinical care in the UK is delivered and monitored according to agreed national guidelines and results are monitored by the National Head and Neck Audit – Data on Head and Neck Oncology (DAHNO). Radiotherapy and surgery are the two treatment modalities used singly or combined for the management of patients with head and neck cancer. Over the past decade there is growing evidence that the use of chemotherapy, molecular and targeted therapy concurrently with radiotherapy achieves a better tumour response and an improvement in patient functional outcome and quality of life survival. The choice of treatment combinations depends on many broad factors: the patients' choice, the site and stage of disease, the expertise of the MDT, and the availability of local facilities.

Early stage tumours

Fewer than 20% of head and neck cancer patients at presentation are in the early stages. The most frequent sites are within the oral cavity, oropharynx and larynx. The treatment of early oral cavity cancer is surgical excision of the primary site with consideration given to treating the neck either by "watch and wait", "sentinel node biopsy" or an elective selective neck dissection. Early tumours of the larynx are most commonly located on the vocal cord or glottic area. In the past, treatment by radiotherapy or surgical excision resulted in similar cure rates but were associated with differing and long-term side-effects. The major effect of treatment in glottic cancer is the effect on the voice quality in the short and long term. The option for surgical excision for small glottic cancers has been improved significantly over the traditional "open technique" by the use of transoral laser excision which has reduced morbidity with minimal effect on the remaining organ function (Figure 24.3). Such advantages have also been demonstrated in early tumours located in the oropharynx – tonsil and posterior tongue.

Advanced tumours

More than 80% of head and neck cancers present at an advanced stage, with approximately 10% manifesting with proven distant metastases, with the highest rate associated with advanced pharyngeal cancer. Recent reports have shown that single modality treatment (surgery or radiotherapy) is associated with poorer

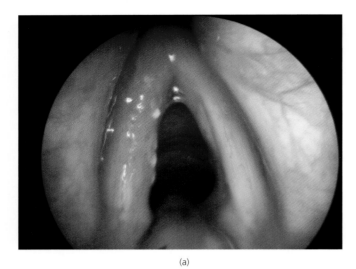

(a)

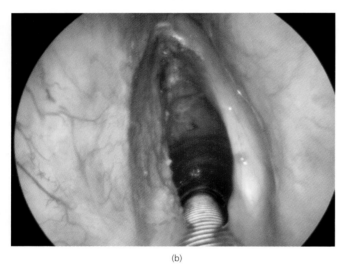

(b)

Figure 24.3 Surgical treatment of an early glottis cancer: (a) pre-laser excision; (b) post-operative view.

outcomes, and prospective randomised studies have shown that combined use of surgery with postoperative radiotherapy, or combined chemoradiotherapy offers the highest chance of achieving a cure.

Surgery

Surgery for head and neck cancers has moved away from major resections with major reconstruction for oropharyngeal and hypopharyngeal cancers, with the exception of oral cavity (Figure 24.4). With the use of endoscopic surgical techniques such as the carbon dioxide laser, employing magnification and the advantages of robotic surgery, more advanced primary stage diseases can be resected without the need for complex flap reconstruction. However, management of the neck disease has remained a choice between surgery in the form of a neck dissection, with postoperative radiotherapy or the use of concurrent chemoradiotherapy. Currently patients who present with significant tumour mass or large volume tumours, usually with significant organ dysfunction such as pain (cartilage destruction), swallowing and breathing difficulties, are more likely to achieve a more rapid relief of symptoms, are likely to have a more prolonged survival, and are more receptive to postoperative treatment such as radiotherapy, for example advanced oral cavity, larynx and hypopharyngeal cancer (Figure 24.5).

Advances have been made in the surgical and radiotherapy techniques used in the treatment of head and neck cancer patients. Minimising the donor morbidity has been achieved by using lower limb flaps with improved functional outcome for oral cavity surgery. The introduction of intensity modulated radiotherapy (IMRT) has allowed for better dose control while at the same time reducing radiation-induced damage to the salivary glands and minimising the resultant xerostomia. The use of chemotherapy has shown in meta-analysis that concomitant chemoradiotherapy (given together) has shown an improvement in locoregional control rates and was associated with a 6.5% increase in survival. The combination of giving chemotherapy with irradiation has also

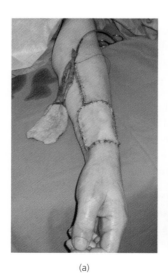

(a)

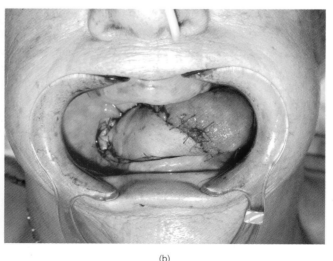

(b)

Figure 24.4 Surgical resection and repair of tongue cancer: (a) radial forearm free flap; (b) repair of surgical defect (hemiglossectomy).

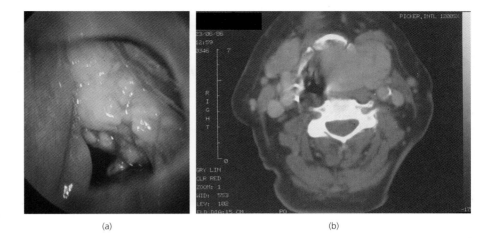

Figure 24.5 Supraglottic cancer (larynx): (a) endoscopic view; (b) CT scan to demonstrate extent of tumour size.

(a)

(b)

shown improvement in the rates of organ conservation, specifically in laryngeal and hypopharyngeal cancers.

Complications and rehabilitation

The treatment of a patient with a head and neck cancer by its nature will result in temporary or permanent functional effects. Some may be life threatening such as aspiration, while other may be cosmetic or result in xerostomia (dry mouth). Surgery by its nature is considered to be the most destructive requiring protracted time in hospital and high risk of post-operative haemorrhage with wound and chest infections. Damage to vital structures such as cranial nerves can affect voice, speech, swallowing and shoulder function permanently. A total laryngectomy will result in patients breathing through a tracheostoma (hole in the neck), loss of voice and alteration swallow (Figure 24.6). Voicing can be achieved by using trachea-oesophageal speech, using a voice prosthesis.

The effects of chemoradiotherapy can be acute or late. Many patients, because of their co-morbidity are not suitable for chemotherapy such as cisplatin, or treatment may be interrupted. Acute complications include neutropoenia, renal toxicity, and mucositis may require urgent readmission to hospital. To ensure adequate nutrition and hydration during treatment the insertion of a gastrostomy may be necessary. However, patients must continue to swallow normally as pharyngeal stenosis is likely to occur which has long-term consequences. Late effects or radiotherapy include soft tissue fibrosis, dysphagia and osteoradionecrosis which may remain for life.

Involvement at the time of diagnosis and involvement of patient treatment planning of speech by language therapists, dietetics, psychologists, pain therapists and many others is very important for the short and long-term management of patients after treatment of their head and neck cancer.

Outcome and survival

Despite improvements in locoregional control for patients with head and neck squamous cell carcinoma, the overall survival has barely changed over the past three decades, considered due to distant metastases. DAHNO 6 (2011), reported patient death within

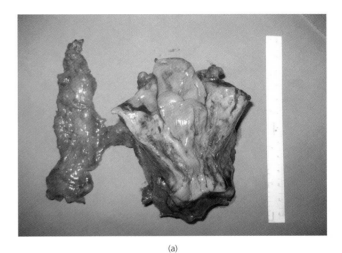

(a)

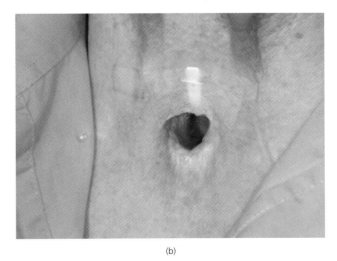

(b)

Figure 24.6 Surgical treatment of advanced laryngeal cancer: (a) total laryngectomy with a neck dissection; (b) late post-operative view of tracheostoma with a trachea-oesophageal voice prosthesis (TEP).

12 months of cancer diagnosis: oral cavity 16.7%, oropharynx 14.1%, larynx 12.1% and hypopharynx 30.6%, suggesting that in order to improve survival, earlier diagnosis is necessary.

Table 24.3 Head and neck cancer survival at 1 and 5 years in England (%).

Site Year	Survival	Oral Cav	OroPx	NasoPx	Larynx	HypoPx	Thyroid	Salivary
1990/92	1 year	72.5	65.62	65.89	82.75	49.10	79.31	76.19
2000/02	1 year	76.89	73.69	74.92	83.03	57.74	88.15	83.23
2004/06	1 year	78.69	79.15	78/45	85.10	58.94	90.07	83.68
1990/92	5 years	49.57	37.03	39.77	64.22	22.29	75.46	58.45
2000/02	5 years	55.95	52.13	49.38	65.26	26.05	80.86	69.33

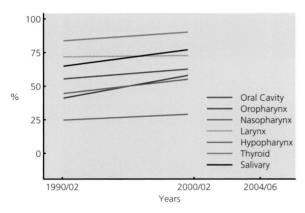

Figure 24.7 Survival for 5 years in England 1990/92 to 2000/02.

The Oxford Cancer Intelligence Unit reported on head and neck cancer patients in England showed a significant trend for improved 1- and 5-year survival figures for years 1990/02 to 2000/02 for all sites (Table 24.3, Figure 24.7). These figures have continued to rise year on year up to 2004/06 when the latest 1-year survival figures only are available: oral cavity 78.69%, oropharynx 79.15%, nasopharynx 78.45%, hypopharynx 58.94%, larynx 85.10%, thyroid 90.07% and salivary gland 83.68% (Figure 24.8).

Management of recurrent or metastatic disease

The overall cure rate for head and neck squamous cell carcinoma is 50%, with locoregional recurrence after treatment being high.

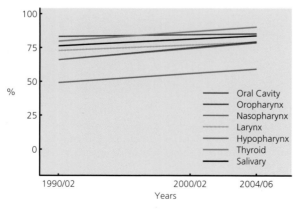

Figure 24.8 Survival for 1 year in England 1990/92 to 2000/06.

Local recurrences are associated with pain, progressive dysphagia, depression, anxiety, fatigue, anorexia and cachexia. The survival after recurrence is months, and for distant metastasis the average is 4 months. Some patients with a locoregional recurrence can be salvaged by surgery or re-irradiation. The majority of patients with recurrent or metastatic disease only qualify for palliative treatment. Treatment choice should be based on factors such as performance status, co-morbidity, prior treatment, symptoms and patient preference. Several of the more traditionally used combination chemotherapy regimens have shown higher response rates but have not affected survival. The addition of cetuximab to the combination of cisplatin or carboplatin and infusional 5-fluorouracil has led to a significant improvement in overall survival in patients with recurrent/metastatic squamous cell carcinaoma of the head and neck. This regimen is recommended for recurrent/metastatic disease patients with good performance status, who otherwise would have been able to tolerate platinum-based combined chemotherapy regimens.

The future

- There is a need to improve public awareness of the association of cigarette smoking and excessive alcohol consumption with head and neck cancer, and that the reduction or avoidance of such social habits would achieve the most significant reduction in the incidence of head and neck cancer, not only in the UK but worldwide. However, there will be a time interval between a public response to reduce smoking and alcohol consumption before the cancer registers will demonstrate any effect.
- In tandem with the above, there is also a need to improve education among public health professionals of the symptoms which may suggest patients who should be referred to specialists to have the diagnosis of head and neck cancer excluded.
- As research has identified more effective molecular or immunotherapy for the treatment of cancer attention must be directed at preventing the development of distant metastases which currently results in many patients who have achieved loco-regional control dying from their disease.

Further reading

Roland NJ, Paleri V (eds). *Head and Neck Cancer: Multidisciplinary Management Guidelines*, 4th edn. ENT UK, London, 2011.
Mehenna H, Jones TM, Gregoire V, Ang KK. Oropharyngeal carcinoma related to human papillomavirus. *BMJ* 2010;**340**:c1439.

Sharma N, Boelaert K, Watkinson JC. Who should treat thyroid cancer? A UK surgical perspective. *Clin Oncol* 2010:**22**;413–18.

Paleri V, Staines K, Sloan P, Douglas A, Wilson J. Evaluation of oral ulceration in primary care. *BMJ* 2010;**340**:c2639.

Mehenna H, Paleri V, West CML, Nutting C. Head and neck cancer – Part 1: Epidemiology, presentation, and prevention. *BMJ* 2010:**341**;c4684.

Mehenna H, West CML, Nutting C, Paleri V. Head and neck cancer – Part 2: Treatment and prognostic factors. *BMJ* 2010:**341**;c4690.

Goh HKC, Ng YK, Teo DTW. Minimal invasive surgery for head and neck cancer. *Lancet Oncol* 2010:**11**;281–86.

Referral guidelines for suspected cancer; Clinical Guidelines 27: Developed by the National Collaborating Institute for Primary Care, June 2005.

Profile of Head and Neck Cancer in England: Incidence, Mortality and Survival. Oxford Cancer Intelligence Unit: January 2010.

National Head and Neck Cancer Audit 2010; The NHS Information Centre, Head and Neck Cancer Audit 2011.

Further resources

Cancerbackup, www.cancerbackup.org.uk

Facial Deformity Charity, www.letsface-it.org.uk

Head and Neck Cancer Charity, www.getahead.org.uk

Mouth Cancer Foundation, www.mouthcancerfoundation.org.uk

National Association of Laryngectomy Clubs, www.nalc.uk.com

Index

Note: Page references in *italics* refer to Figures; those in **bold** refer to Tables

ABC of Pain

Lesley A. Colvin & Marie Fallon
Western General Hospital, Edinburgh; University of Edinburgh

Pain is a common presentation and this brand new title focuses on the pain management issues most often encountered in primary care. *ABC of Pain*:

- Covers all the chronic pain presentations in primary care right through to tertiary and palliative care and includes guidance on pain management in special groups such as pregnancy, children, the elderly and the terminally ill
- Includes new findings on the effectiveness of interventions and the progression to acute pain and appropriate pharmacological management
- Features pain assessment, epidemiology and the evidence base in a truly comprehensive reference
- Provides a global perspective with an international list of expert contributors

JUNE 2012 | 9781405176217 | 128 PAGES | £24.99/US$44.95/€32.90/AU$47.95

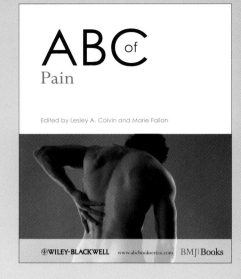

ABC of Urology

3RD EDITION

Chris Dawson & Janine Nethercliffe
Fitzwilliam Hospital, Peterborough; Edith Cavell Hospital, Peterborough

Urological conditions are common, accounting for up to one third of all surgical admissions to hospital. Outside of hospital care urological problems are a common reason for patients needing to see their GP.

- *ABC of Urology, 3rd Edition* provides a comprehensive overview of urology
- Focuses on the diagnosis and management of the most common urological conditions
- Features 4 additional chapters: improved coverage of renal and testis cancer in separate chapters and new chapters on management of haematuria, laparoscopy, trauma and new urological advances
- Ideal for GPs and trainee GPs, and is useful for junior doctors undergoing surgical training, while medical students and nurses undertaking a urological placement as part of their training programme will find this edition indispensable

MARCH 2012 | 9780470657171 | 88 PAGES | £23.99/US$37.95/€30.90/AU$47.95

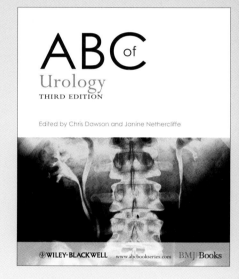

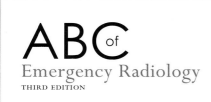

ABC of Emergency Radiology

3RD EDITION

Otto Chan
London Independent Hospital

The *ABC of Emergency Radiology, 3rd Edition* an invaluable resource for accident and emergency staff, trainee radiologists, medical students, nurses, radiographers and all medical personnel involved in the immediate care of trauma patients.

- Follows a systematic approach to assessing radiographs
- Each chapter covers a different part of the body, leading through the anatomy for ease of use
- Includes clear explanations and instructions on the appearances of radiological abnormalities with comparison to normal radiographs throughout
- Incorporates over 400 radiographs

JANUARY 2013 | 9780470670934 | 144 PAGES | £29.99/US$48.95/€38.90/AU$57.95

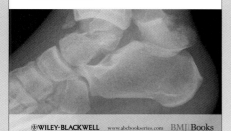

ABC of Resuscitation

6TH EDITION

Jasmeet Soar, Gavin D. Perkins & Jerry Nolan
Southmead Hospital, Bristol; University of Warwick, Coventry; Royal United Hospital, Bath

A practical guide to the latest resuscitation advice for the non-specialist *ABC of Resuscitation, 6th Edition*:

- Covers the core knowledge on the management of patients with cardiopulmonary arrest
- Includes the 2010 European Resuscitation Council Guidelines for Resuscitation
- Edited by specialists responsible for producing the European and UK 2010 resuscitation guidelines

DECEMBER 2012 | 9780470672594| 144 PAGES | £28.99/US$47.95/€37.90/AU$54.95

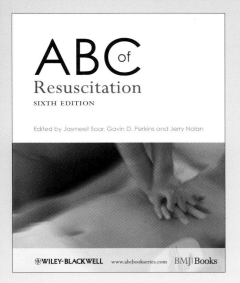

ABC_{of} ABC of Epilepsy

W. Henry Smithson & Matthew C. Walker
University of Sheffield; University College London

In the new, easy to navigate ABC series format *ABC of Epilepsy*:

* Provides a practical guide for general practitioners, and all those working in primary care
* Includes the diagnosis, treatment and management of epilepsy, and for the continued monitoring and long term support
* Covers anti-epileptic drugs and non-drug treatments, as well as self-management and living with epilepsy
* Highly illustrated throughout to clearly present what epilepsy is, its classification, and how to diagnose it

MARCH 2012 | 9781444333985 | 48 PAGES | £19.99/US$33.95/€25.90/AU$37.95

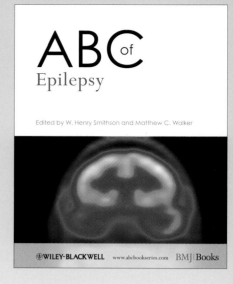

ABC_{of} Prostate Cancer

Prokar Dasgupta & Roger Kirby
Guys & St Thomas' Hospitals, London; The Prostate Centre, London

Prostate cancer is the most common cancer in men in the UK and US and the second most common worldwide. *ABC of Prostate Cancer*:

* Provides fully illustrated guidance on the treatment and management of prostate cancer
* Covers the biology, anatomy, and pathology of prostate cancer, screening, and active surveillance and monitoring
* Presents an assessment of treatment options including prostatectomy, bracytherapy, chemotherapy and immunotherapy, along with modern diagnostic tests and an overview of new approaches to prostate cancer
* With an international author team, *ABC of Prostate Cancer* is ideal for GPs, family physicians, specialist nurses, junior doctors, medical students and others working with prostate cancer patients and their families

DECEMBER 2011 | 9781444334371 | 80 PAGES | £22.99/US$35.95/€39.95/AU$44.95

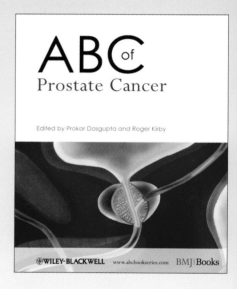

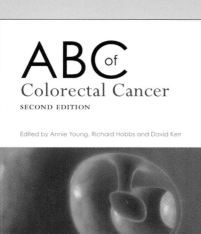

ABCof Colorectal Cancer

2ND EDITION

Annie Young, Richard Hobbs & David Kerr
University of Warwick; University of Oxford; University of Oxford

Colorectal cancer is the third most common cancer in men and the second most common cancer in women worldwide. The second edition to this practical guide:

- Provides an invaluable guide for the non-specialist on the diagnosis and treatment of colorectal cancer and is ideal for GPs, junior doctors, nurses and allied health professionals
- Covers core knowledge on therapy, management, and supportive care interventions, diagnosis follow up and advanced and innovative treatment and highlights the evidence base throughout
- Includes key information on new drug treatments and the new UK screening program and guidelines
- Maps the "real life" treatment pathway to enhance the resources' practical use

NOVEMBER 2011 | 9781405177634 | 88 PAGES | £19.99/US$30.95/€25.90/AU$37.95

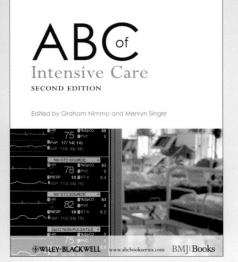

ABCof Intensive Care

2ND EDITION

Graham R. Nimmo & Mervyn Singer
Western General Hospital, Edinburgh; University College London

Intensive care is an increasingly important medical specialty and has a strong multidisciplinary component with a common stem for initial training.

This practical guide to intensive care:

- Provides the core knowledge of intensive care patient management with best practice management in the intensive care unit
- Covers topics from general principles through to critical care outreach and end of life care, key organ system support, monitoring, sepsis, brain-stem death, and nutrition in intensive care and organ donation
- References key evidence, and further reading and resources for comprehensive coverage in each chapter
- Is endorsed by the Intensive Care Society
- Is ideal for junior doctors, medical students and specialist nurses working in an acute hospital setting and for anyone involved in the management and care of intensive care patients

SEPTEMBER 2011 | 9781405178037 | 88 PAGES | £19.99/US$30.95/€25.90/AU$37.95

ALSO AVAILABLE

ABC of Adolescence
Russell Viner
2005 | 9780727915740 | 56 PAGES
£26.99 / US$41.95 / €34.90 / AU$52.95

ABC of Antithrombotic Therapy
Gregory Y. H. Lip & Andrew D. Blann
2003 | 9780727917713 | 67 PAGES
£26.50 / US$41.95 / €34.90 / AU$52.95

ABC of Arterial and Venous Disease, 2nd Edition
Richard Donnelly & Nick J. M. London
2009 | 9781405178891 | 120 PAGES
£31.50 / US$54.95 / €40.90 / AU$59.95

ABC of Asthma, 6th Edition
John Rees, Dipak Kanabar & Shriti Pattani
2009 | 9781405185967 | 104 PAGES
£26.99 / US$41.95 / €34.90 / AU$52.95

ABC of Burns
Shehan Hettiaratchy, Remo Papini & Peter Dziewulski
2004 | 9780727917874 | 56 PAGES
£26.50 / US$41.95 / €34.90 / AU$52.95

ABC of Child Protection, 4th Edition
Roy Meadow, Jacqueline Mok & Donna Rosenberg
2007 | 9780727918178 | 120 PAGES
£35.50 / US$59.95 / €45.90 / AU$67.95

ABC of Clinical Electrocardiography, 2nd Edition
Francis Morris, William J. Brady & John Camm
2008 | 9781405170642 | 112 PAGES
£34.50 / US$57.95 / €44.90 / AU$67.95

ABC of Clinical Genetics, 3rd Edition
Helen M. Kingston
2002 | 9780727916273 | 120 PAGES
£34.50 / US$57.95 / €44.90 / AU$67.95

ABC of Clinical Haematology, 3rd Edition
Drew Provan
2007 | 9781405153539 | 112 PAGES
£34.50 / US$59.95 / €44.90 / AU$67.95

ABC of Clinical Leadership
Tim Swanwick & Judy McKimm
2010 | 9781405198172 | 88 PAGES
£20.95 / US$32.95 / €26.90 / AU$39.95

ABC of Complementary Medicine, 2nd Edition
Catherine Zollman, Andrew J. Vickers & Janet Richardson
2008 | 9781405136570 | 64 PAGES
£28.95 / US$47.95 / €37.90 / AU$54.95

ABC of COPD, 2nd Edition
Graeme P. Currie
2010 | 9781444333886 | 88 PAGES
£23.95 / US$37.95 / €30.90 / AU$47.95

ABC of Dermatology, 5th Edition
Paul K. Buxton & Rachael Morris-Jones
2009 | 9781405170659 | 224 PAGES
£34.50 / US$58.95 / €44.90 / AU$67.95

ABC of Diabetes, 6th Edition
Tim Holt & Sudhesh Kumar
2007 | 9781405177849 | 112 PAGES
£31.50 / US$52.95 / €40.90 / AU$59.95

ABC of Eating Disorders
Jane Morris
2008 | 9780727918437 | 80 PAGES
£26.50 / US$41.95 / €34.90 / AU$52.95

ABC of Emergency Differential Diagnosis
Francis Morris & Alan Fletcher
2009 | 9781405170635 | 96 PAGES
£31.50 / US$55.95 / €40.90 / AU$59.95

ABC of Geriatric Medicine
Nicola Cooper, Kirsty Forrest & Graham Mulley
2009 | 9781405169424 | 88 PAGES
£26.50 / US$44.95 / €34.90 / AU$52.95

ABC of Headache
Anne MacGregor & Alison Frith
2008 | 9781405170666 | 88 PAGES
£23.95 / US$41.95 / €30.90 / AU$47.95

ABC of Heart Failure, 2nd Edition
Russell C. Davis, Michael K. Davis & Gregory Y. H. Lip
2006 | 9780727916440 | 72 PAGES
£26.50 / US$41.95 / €34.90 / AU$52.95

ABC of Imaging in Trauma
Leonard J. King & David C. Wherry
2008 | 9781405183321 | 144 PAGES
£31.50 / US$50.95 / €40.90 / AU$59.95

ABC of Interventional Cardiology, 2nd Edition
Ever D. Grech
2010 | 9781405170673 | 120 PAGES
£25.95 / US$40.95 / €33.90 / AU$49.95

ABC of Learning and Teaching in Medicine, 2nd Edition
Peter Cantillon & Diana Wood
2009 | 9781405185974 | 96 PAGES
£22.99 / US$35.95 / €29.90 / AU$44.95

ABC of Liver, Pancreas and Gall Bladder
Ian Beckingham
1905 | 9780727915313 | 64 PAGES
£24.95 / US$39.95 / €32.90 / AU$47.95

ABC of Lung Cancer
Ian Hunt, Martin M. Muers & Tom Treasure
2009 | 9781405146524 | 64 PAGES
£25.95 / US$41.95 / €33.90 / AU$49.95

ABC of Medical Law
Lorraine Corfield, Ingrid Granne & William Latimer-Sayer
2009 | 9781405176286 | 64 PAGES
£24.95 / US$39.95 / €32.90 / AU$47.95

ABC of Mental Health, 2nd Edition
Teifion Davies & Tom Craig
2009 | 9780727916396 | 128 PAGES
£32.50 / US$52.95 / €41.90 / AU$62.95

ABC of Obesity
Naveed Sattar & Mike Lean
2007 | 9781405136747 | 64 PAGES
£24.99 / US$39.99 / €32.90 / AU$47.95

ABC of One to Seven, 5th Edition
Bernard Valman
2009 | 9781405181051 | 168 PAGES
£32.50 / US$52.95 / €41.90 / AU$62.95

ABC of Palliative Care, 2nd Edition
Marie Fallon & Geoffrey Hanks
2006 | 9781405130790 | 96 PAGES
£30.50 / US$52.95 / €39.90 / AU$57.95

ABC of Patient Safety
John Sandars & Gary Cook
2007 | 9781405156929 | 64 PAGES
£28.50 / US$46.99 / €36.90 / AU$54.95

ABC of Practical Procedures
Tim Nutbeam & Ron Daniels
2009 | 9781405185950 | 144 PAGES
£31.50 / US$50.95 / €40.90 / AU$59.95

ABC of Preterm Birth
William McGuire & Peter Fowlie
2005 | 9780727917638 | 56 PAGES
£26.50 / US$41.95 / €34.90 / AU$52.95

ABC of Psychological Medicine
Richard Mayou, Michael Sharpe & Alan Carson
2003 | 9780727915566 | 72 PAGES
£26.99 / US$41.95 / €34.90 / AU$52.95

ABC of Rheumatology, 4th Edition
Ade Adebajo
2009 | 9781405170680 | 192 PAGES
£31.95 / US$50.95 / €41.90 / AU$62.95

ABC of Sepsis
Ron Daniels & Tim Nutbeam
2009 | 9781405181945 | 104 PAGES
£31.50 / US$52.95 / €40.90 / AU$59.95

ABC of Sexual Health, 2nd Edition
John Tomlinson
2004 | 9780727917591 | 96 PAGES
£31.50 / US$52.95 / €40.90 / AU$59.95

ABC of Skin Cancer
Sajjad Rajpar & Jerry Marsden
2008 | 9781405162197 | 80 PAGES
£26.50 / US$47.95 / €34.90 / AU$52.95

ABC of Spinal Disorders
Andrew Clarke, Alwyn Jones & Michael O'Malley
2009 | 9781405170697 | 72 PAGES
£24.95 / US$39.95 / €32.90 / AU$47.95

ABC of Sports and Exercise Medicine, 3rd Edition
Gregory Whyte, Mark Harries & Clyde Williams
2005 | 9780727918130 | 136 PAGES
£34.95 / US$62.95 / €44.90 / AU$67.95

ABC of Subfertility
Peter Braude & Alison Taylor
2005 | 9780727915344 | 64 PAGES
£24.95 / US$39.95 / €32.90 / AU$47.95

ABC of the First Year, 6th Edition
Bernard Valman & Roslyn Thomas
2009 | 9781405180375 | 136 PAGES
£31.50 / US$55.95 / €40.90 / AU$59.95

ABC of the Upper Gastrointestinal Tract
Robert Logan, Adam Harris & J. J. Misiewicz
2002 | 9780727912664 | 54 PAGES
£26.50 / US$41.95 / €34.90 / AU$52.95

ABC of Transfusion, 4th Edition
Marcela Contreras
2009 | 9781405156462 | 128 PAGES
£31.50 / US$55.95 / €40.90 / AU$59.95

ABC of Tubes, Drains, Lines and Frames
Adam Brooks, Peter F. Mahoney & Brian Rowlands
2008 | 9781405160148 | 88 PAGES
£26.50 / US$41.95 / €34.90 / AU$52.95